"This is a call-to-arms for those living with multiple sclerosis to take control of their lives and be empowered by someone living with MS. Stachowiak (author of the MS pages on About.com) takes the reader through the basics of the condition, outlining what types of MS there are and the symptoms, treatment, and professional care available. She blends that information with the practical and sometimes intangible aspects of emotional health and enjoying life. With a conversational but authoritative voice, this a positive joy to read and work through."
—*Library Journal*

"Intelligent, empowering, and realistic are just some of the words that describe Julie Stachowiak's book, Multiple Sclerosis Manifesto. A person living with MS, an epidemiologist, an advocate, and a writer for ms.about.com, Julie Stachowiak knows all too well the emotional and physical struggles MS can bring to daily life. Armed with many years of knowledge and firsthand expertise, Stachowiak has, in her book, put together a wonderful testament to coping with MS.

... honest, straightforward, and at times humorous, Stachowiak offers practical advice about the many obstacles one will inevitably encounter while living with a chronic illness...Chapters are easy to read, but it's Stachowiak's unique writing style, knowledge, and carefully thought-out presentation of the material that makes navigating through the pages simple and thoroughly enjoyable."
—*MSFocus*

"In addition to its informational content, the principal merit of the book by Stachowiak is the ability to hold the reader's attention... A newly diagnosed person with MS who is shocked and feels fully unaware of what to expect will find the book very valuable, since it can reach and fill the person's heart with the will to win...

[Stachowiak] makes good use of both the popular language writing and indispensable medical science terms to express her point of view and approach infinite issues arising in the course of the disease. Oftentimes, these seemingly insignificant issues are ignored by professionals and writers of other guidances and papers, because it requires an aspect of personal experience and understanding of the situation... the book reveals that MS is no end of life but merely another period of life with a more complex strategy...The book gets the reader engaged as compared to distant advices found in MS editions of the kind... she sends a message of positivism and audacity to 'live with it.'"
—*MSCare.org*

The Multiple Sclerosis Manifesto

The Multiple Sclerosis Manifesto

Action to Take, Principles to Live By

Julie Stachowiak, PhD

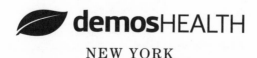

NEW YORK

Library of Congress Cataloging-in-Publication Data

Stachowiak, Julie.
     The multiple sclerosis manifesto : action to take, principles to live by / Julie Stachowiak.
        p. cm.
     Includes bibliographical references and index.
     ISBN 978-1-932603-44-6 (pbk.)
     1. Multiple sclerosis—Popular works. I. Title.
     RC377.S725 2010
     616.8'34—dc22   2009041458

Made in the United States of America

10 11 12   5 4 3 2

To my readers with MS and those who love them.
Take care of yourselves, my friends.

Contents

Acknowledgements

For a very long time, I have wanted to write a book. I just didn't think I could do a good job. After being diagnosed with multiple sclerosis, I had to live with this disease. I didn't think I could do a good job at that, either. I've now done both things, and I'm feeling pretty good about how I handled them. It would have been a much different story if I had to do them alone.

First, I want to thank the readers of ms.about.com. People from all over the world, with all different kinds of symptoms and disabilities write to me and tell me that I am helping them with my words. I truly appreciate that, and it was the motivation to write this book. I also appreciate the people that write in to tell me that I am wrong, that I don't know what I am talking about and that I have done a crappy job of explaining something. These people clearly have passion, they are engaged with the world and they care enough to respond to things that they don't like. After I lick my wounds from some of their comments, I can usually find the lesson in their criticism. I also am grateful to my new friends at a certain MS forum (you know who you are) for providing a place to "rest" from it all.

I am equally grateful to About.com for giving me the opportunity to reach as many people with multiple sclerosis as I do. I want to thank my editor, Joy Victory, for giving me a long editorial leash and allowing me to develop my voice, while encouraging me the whole time. The Medical Director of About.com, Dr. Kate Grossman, has provided amazing direction and held high standards, always thinking about how the readers will be helped by what they encounter on our pages. The fact that these people and others at About.com are now my friends makes the work fun.

Thank you to Noreen Henson at Demos Health Publishing for encouraging me to "tell it like it is" and for pulling my innermost feelings out into the light, so that other people living with multiple sclerosis can see that they are not alone in their fight. Thank you for making me laugh. I would also like to thank the rest of the staff of Demos for believing in this project and doing all the stuff that goes into making a book that is rarely seen or acknowledged.

I would also like to thank my former professors and colleagues at the Johns Hopkins Bloomberg School of Public Health, people who embrace the idea that health is both an individual matter and a societal right. It was at Hopkins that I really learned how to get to the meat of a study and ask "how will this help anyone?" as well as tear apart false assumptions about "patients" and "the chronically ill." These skills have served me well since I have actually become one of those people about whom assumptions are made. The science at Hopkins is spectacular, made more so by the fact that the humans being studied remain humans to the scientists. I would especially like to thank my former advisor, Dr. Chris Beyrer, who always encouraged me to "speak truth," even when it was neither convenient nor comfortable to do so.

The staff of AIDS infoshare Russia has been an inspiration to everything I do since we formed the organization in 1993. The degree of their resourcefulness in the face of adversity is always a true inspiration to me in my darkest hours. Specifically, I would like to thank Stanislav Erastov, Victor Lazarev, Vladimir Mogilnii and Katya Medvedovskaya for showing me how to get things done. Of course, my closest friend, Alena Peryshkina, has always been a beacon to me as she successfully holds things together for her family, her organization and her country. I love you, Lena.

There are those of you who have reached out during the writing of this book to check in with me, often throwing a lifeline of a laugh or a pep talk when most needed. My thanks to: Ingrid Monroy, Leslie Lakes, Whitney Bishop, Rebecca Kendall, Anne Dadura, Penny Khuri, Lynn Crowe and many others who define the word "friend." I especially want to thank Bridget Riha, without whom this book writing endeavor would have been much lonelier and much, much less fun. Thank you for laughing out loud when I needed you to, and holding my hand while I pounded my virtual head against the virtual wall when the words wouldn't come.

To my neurologist (the good one), Dr. Rivera, and all of his staff at Maxine Mesinger Multiple Sclerosis Clinic, for giving me the example of what a patient should strive for in his or her quest for a great partnership in his or her medical care.

Lastly, I want to thank my family. I thank my mother-in-law, Paula, for keeping the house (and the twins) sane during the times when I wrote to the point of near insanity. I thank Janelle (MamMaw) and Annie (Nannie) for giving me the safe haven that I needed to let my hair down, put my feet up and let my neurons "reconnect" in peace. I thank my dad and my brother for asking about me in the heat of the summer when they knew it might make me weepy.

Above all, I thank my husband for pretty much everything and my twins for being patient when Mommy was writing her words. I love you.

Introduction: The Manifesto

This is a book about dignity.

More specifically, this book is about living with dignity while simultaneously dealing with multiple sclerosis, a disease that can eradicate our sense of control and our self-esteem if we are not actively fighting to keep ourselves whole every moment.

Dignity is about quality of life, which can be defined as "the degree to which a person enjoys the important possibilities of his or her life," the definition used by the Quality of Life Research Unit of the University of Toronto. To that end, *The Multiple Sclerosis Manifesto* will take you through different aspects of life with MS, in search of ways to increase the possibilities of your life. These include optimizing medical care and managing symptoms, but also extend to relationships, emotions, activism, and much more. In each of these areas, *The Multiple Sclerosis Manifesto* will help you to figure out what you need, identify opportunities, understand the challenges, and get your needs met. Your personal MS Manifesto is your commitment to exploring and developing the possibilities of your life. It's all about the principles and rules you will create to guide the next phase of your life.

Each Person's MS Is Personal

We know that there are four different types of MS. To complicate matters, even within the different types, we all have different symptoms. Even among people sharing a symptom, the spectrum is huge—one person's spasticity results in being wheelchair-bound, while another person notices only that it is more difficult to navigate stairs on some days.

Despite these differences, there are things that make us similar to other people living with MS. We can't say for sure what the future holds. We really don't know what our next symptom will be or when it will show up. We don't know which medications or procedures will help us feel better until we try them.

We do know that we didn't do anything to cause the MS. And, sadly, we also know that, for the moment, there is no cure for MS. Most of all, we know that we would really rather not have MS.

For People with MS, by a Person with MS

As a person who is living with MS, some days more successfully than others, I have made it my mission to share with you what has worked to keep me going, to keep me from losing my confidence, and to preserve those parts of myself that I take pride in. After my diagnosis and before becoming the Guide to MS at About.com, I searched for information that would help me to understand what was going on with both my body and mind, as well as make me feel understood. I mostly found information written by "experts" who discussed what MS "patients" *should* do. I also turned up other writings by people with MS who rhapsodized about the wonderful advances in treatment and touted the power of a positive attitude.

> ### The Real World
> Okay, multiple sclerosis sucks. It truly does. Let's just get that out there.

Only rarely did I run across something that spoke to me, written by someone who said, "Yep, MS is crappy, no doubt about it. This is what I tried that made it a little less crappy for awhile." Usually I found these people in the world of blogs, telling their stories to a limited audience composed of their loved ones and like-minded MSers whom they collected along the way.

When I began writing for About.com, I just wanted to write about things as I saw them. I wanted to "speak truth" about multiple sclerosis, to decode some of the mysteries of MS for whoever might be interested, and to reap the therapeutic value I found in indulging myself in this personal subject. I was unprepared for the responses that I got. I have run the gamut of emotions and discovered new depths of feeling when someone tells me that her doctor laughed at the idea that MS can cause pain or that his sister accused him of causing his MS by smoking pot a couple of times in college. I was stunned that others felt such a sense of isolation and of being misunderstood that they chose to hide their symptoms from their closest family members just to "fit in." I cried (and still do) when people write to me about the people that they will never become, the dreams that they have left behind, the dignity that has been stolen from them.

However, there are glimmers—and even rays—of hope and forti-tude, as well. People tell me that they show something to their doctors and insist that a new therapy be tried. Others rejoice to find out some-thing that was torturing them is a symptom of MS and that there is something that *might* work, just *might* help them feel better. I am mostly humbled by the people who simply tell me "thank you," as I am the one who is grateful to have this opportunity to communicate with people, many of whom are much braver and much stronger than I about this whole MS thing.

My Manifesto

Back in my 20s, I knew absolutely *everything* about how the world should work and how people should behave. You would have loved me, I'm sure, as I tried to get you to quit your day job and leave your families to help Russian orphans, homeless people with HIV, heroin addicts, victims of the Holocaust, women who had suffered botched abortions, and anybody who just seemed kind of sad. Those of you brave enough to tell me that these weren't your issues or that these problems didn't directly touch your lives would have had the chance to snicker to yourself (or laugh in my face) when I quoted the ancient Greek historian, Thucydides, proclaiming that "Justice will not come to Athens until those who are not injured are as indignant as those who are injured." I bet I was just precious.

Then lots of years went by and lots of stuff happened—now I'm in my 40s and I have multiple sclerosis.

Many years of life in the real world have enlightened the once-fervent advocate of "rightness" that I used to be. For instance, I learned that it wasn't prudent to rush into making bold statements without researching all sides of the issue and finding middle ground. I know that bad behavior toward me usually has its roots in someone's insecurity or lack of maturity and that I should forgive these transgressions and be the bigger person. Many people have felt the need to point out the fact I am "lucky" that I *only* have MS, since other people have things that are much worse.

Screw all that.
Here is my manifesto.
I will . . .

- Scratch my itchy injection sites with abandon—if you don't like it, don't look.

- Try not to fly into a rage when someone asks me how long I have left or if I am one of Jerry's Kids, but I will firmly educate them about MS in a way they probably won't forget.

- Open my arms to anyone who tells me that they have just been diagnosed with MS or may possibly have MS and just listen, without lying about everything being okay and without doing a "reality dump" of all the things about MS that are not okay.

- Remember that if a potential side effect freaks me out, I probably shouldn't take that drug, as the anxiety would outweigh any benefit I might get.

- Never compare myself to others—not to engage in self-pity that someone else is healthier than I and not to reassure myself that I am not as bad off as someone else. Either comparison makes me feel dirty somehow.

- Take my child who has just shouted, "Mommy, look! A man in a wheelchair!" by the hand and introduce her to the man (rather than shushing her), and teach her that the man in the wheelchair might be very nice or he might be a nasty son of a bitch, and that the wheelchair is immaterial to who someone is.

- Someday actually *do* it—slowly, *very* slowly make my way across a finish line somewhere, wearing my T-shirt that says "I have MS" on the front and "So why are you behind me?" on the back.

- Kiss my husband on the spot behind his left ear that always smells good and tell him that I love him, knowing that the bullshit that comes with my MS has made him sigh a little more deeply and watch over me a little more closely as we go through life together.

Those are the things that I will do to get through this.

The Bigger Picture

You also have things that you will do to navigate your own road with MS. It is a journey that none of us signed up for, but that we find ourselves taking nonetheless. So let's think about this strategically, both as individuals and as a group. What can we do to make the hard parts easier and the good parts last longer? How can we make sure that our actions help us, but also make a difference for those who have similar challenges—what can we do to make our efforts "stick" longer?

I've presented my ideas in the book to give you some guidance in "getting to better" in your own life, but also some reassurance that you are not alone in this thing. There are others out there—many of us. Our efforts can be synergistic: if we can figure this out, we can be a mighty force to bring long-needed changes to our world—whether the result is a more convenient ramp at your neighborhood bank or the president putting his pen to a new piece of legislation, we can make these things happen. Don't doubt it for a minute.

1

Proceed with Confidence

When I was little, I had a number of aspirations for what and whom I wanted to be when I grew up:

I wanted to be a cocktail waitress—loved the outfit.

I wanted to be a ballerina—again, the outfit.

I wanted to be a veterinarian, until I was turned off by the whole "putting to sleep" thing.

I wanted to be a photographer and actually went down this path all the way to college, only to have my potential career cut short by an allergy to photographic chemicals that forced me to change majors.

I am only including the least embarrassing examples in what was a huge, long list—many have been forgotten. While I was entertaining the thoughts of each of these career paths, it never crossed my mind that I would somehow lack the skills or be unable to achieve my goals. In my mind I *was* that ballerina or that veterinarian. I always knew where I was going, even if it periodically changed radically.

Despite the varied list and the fact that many of the other careers that I once felt were my destiny now escape my memory, I am absolutely, 100% sure that I never aspired to be "a person with multiple sclerosis." All the same, here I am, a person with multiple sclerosis. And, my friend, here you are, too.

Take Charge

You are in charge of how you react to your MS.

So, what do we do with this MS component of our identities? We can take a number of paths. We can be people with MS who "didn't deserve it," who had brilliant careers as [fill in the blank] cut short, who struggle every day with thoughts of what might have been. We can be defined by our symptoms, angry when they interfere with our lives and terrified about how much worse they might get. We can compare ourselves to others who don't live with a chronic illness and wonder why it was us, of all people, who have to factor the unknowns of MS into our futures. Although all of those versions of ourselves might be accurate at different times, we probably don't want them to be included in the vision of who we are striving to be. For myself, I want to be a person with MS who is moving forward, not shrinking back, despite fears and uncertainty—I'll be bold enough to say that I want that for you, too.

Take Charge

Commit yourself to being the person you want to be.

To do something well, we need to be committed. It needs to be our identity. We need to be convinced that we are or will become who we aspire to be. That conviction is how we get there. That is how I will become the person with MS who is not standing still.

Do Your Best

Build your confidence to attain the dignity, peace, and happiness that you deserve. Be proud of yourself.

This chapter is about confidence. Confidence is a large part of dignity and inner peace. Confidence is also one of the most difficult things to find and hold on to when living with a changing chronic disease. Ask yourself—how different would your life be if you faced your MS with calm assurance and felt in control? Confidence comes from inside, from always knowing where one is going, even if it changes. It is having an identity that you are proud of, both as a guiding tool for your own actions as well as an image that you present to others.

Develop Your Personal Mission Statement

A mission statement is a brief description of the fundamental purpose of a business or organization. These institutions create mission statements to help focus their efforts and prevent things from getting too chaotic and diffuse when confronted with internal problems or external challenges. Basically, mission statements are designed to keep the company or organization on track so that it can achieve its goals. Even as an individual trying to maneuver my way through life without the "noise" of a whole organization to worry about, I know that I am in perpetual need of a bigger vision to keep me looking up and moving forward, and to prevent me from getting too tangled up in the challenges that come along daily.

Some examples of mission statements from businesses or organizations include:

"The mission of the National Multiple Sclerosis Society is to end the devastating effects of MS."

"The mission of Yale College is to seek exceptionally promising students of all backgrounds from across the nation and around the world and to educate them, through mental discipline and social experience, to develop their intellectual, moral, civic and creative capacities to the fullest. The aim of this education is the cultivation of citizens with a rich awareness of our human heritage to lead and serve in every sphere of human activity."

My all-time favorite, just for the sheer *chutzpah* of it, comes from the Microsoft Corporation, which changed its mission statement from "To empower people through great software—any time, any place, and on any device" to "To enable people and businesses throughout the world to realize their full potential."

Writing a mission statement for yourself will help you become more determined and focused on what you want to do and who you want to be, as well as define how your MS fits into these plans.

Take Charge

To be in control, you need to know where you are going. Create your personal mission statement today.

Here are the steps to writing your own personal mission statement:

Define yourself. The first step of your mission statement is to define who is writing it. You could use your name, followed by a description of the roles most important to you as well as some of the things that you really enjoy.

I'll try out my example on you: *"I, Julie Stachowiak, am a wife, a mother, an epidemiologist, and a writer, who loves reading, cooking, and learning new things."*

What you put in your statement is up to you—you should include the things that are most essential to you own sense of self.

Write your dedication statement. Next, you will list what you are dedicated to—the things you are trying to accomplish in your life. Your statement defines what you aspire to be. It contains your values and motivates you to stick with your plans.

In my example, I might decide: *"I am dedicated to creating a safe and happy home for my family and enjoying the beautiful and delicious things life has to offer."*

Mention your MS. Because you have MS, and it will play some part in your life, it is important to include that in your mission statement. You can write that you "happen to have" multiple sclerosis. So my statement continues with, *"I happen to have MS."*

Then, put your MS in its place. This is where you "lay down the law" to your MS. You put limits on your MS and how it affects both your role and dedication to living in accord with your values and your goals.

In my case I wrote: *"but MS won't impact the happiness in my family or stop me from doing the things that I love."*

State your strategy. You can then outline what actions you are going to take to become the person who you aspire to be, as well as how you are going to apply your personal ideals and ethics to living your life. This is especially important for those times when things are turned upside-down and you are trying to juggle stressful situations. List the actions that you are taking to manage your MS and its symptoms, to keep your attitude and energy high, and to live the life that you desire. Be very specific. The more details you include, the more powerful your mission statement will be. I wrote: *"because I am going to monitor my symptoms closely, pursue the most effective treatment that I can find (even if it takes some trial and error), try to live in the moment, and not let stress or the fear of this damn illness impact my happiness."*

Put it all together. Putting all of my statements together, I now have the following mission statement: *"I, Julie Stachowiak, am a wife, a mother, an epidemiologist, and a writer, who loves reading, cooking, and learning new things. I am dedicated to creating a safe and happy home for my family and enjoying the beautiful and delicious things life has to offer. I happen to have MS, but it won't impact the happiness in my family or stop me from doing the things that I love, because I am going to monitor my symptoms closely, pursue the most effective treatment that I can find (even if it takes some trial and error), try to live in the moment, and not let stress or the fear of this damn illness impact my happiness."*

Repeat this daily for a week. Writing the mission statement once will probably give you something that is good; however, reviewing your statement and thinking about it daily for a week will create a useful and meaningful mission statement for you. That is your goal. It may sound excessive, but repeat this exercise seven days in a row. You don't have to spend a lot of time each day, but coming back to your statement seven times will help you to refine the language and make the statement fit your life perfectly. Just spend five or ten minutes tweaking the language, making sure you include everything and honing the overall message of your mission statement.

Do it your way. Don't worry about grammar. No one is going to read your mission statement—the only person it needs to speak to is you. Feel free to change the format of your mission statement if something else will work better for you. You can add extra statements or put in bullet points. Do anything that works for you when creating your statement.

The Real World

If you don't know where you want to go in life, no one can help you get there (including yourself).

Stick it on the fridge. When you are finished, place your mission statement in a place where you can see it every day. Be proud of it and link everything you do to making it a reality.

Ask for input (if you want). Your friends and family may be able to help you create the right language and ideas to include in your mission statement. They can also give you feedback on how well it describes you and might think of things that you have left out.

Be realistic. Only include things that you plan to do or have the desire to achieve. This isn't a wish list, but a strategic vision to guide your actions. Your goal should be to strive to make each component in your statement a reality.

Start today. Don't wait. Just jot down notes. Don't worry about editing or putting things in full sentences. Get your wheels turning on this.

Take it further. Turn your mission statement into a plan. Take each of the items and write about how you will achieve them. Make lists of the steps you need to take. Take these lists and prioritize the items. Create for yourself a comprehensive plan to manage your illness and achieve the life you describe in your mission statement.

Now that your personal mission statement defines what you want to do and who you want to be, let's figure out how to make it happen.

Self-Efficacy is Your Best Weapon Against this Disease

Henry Ford is quoted as saying, "Whether you think you can or think you can't, you're right."[1] He was talking about self-efficacy, a person's belief that he or she is able to reach his or her goals. Self-efficacy is a concept that psychologists have studied for decades and has been linked to successful coping with chronic illness. Self-efficacy comes from different sources. By paying attention to and capitalizing on those situations where we can gain self-efficacy, we can actually create the confidence that is so crucial to getting what we want and need.

Do Your Best
Think you can and you probably will.

Here is the formula to build up a healthy sense of self-efficacy:

Experience repeated success. The most important contributor to a person's self-efficacy is his or her success—if someone succeeds, especially in situations where he has had to overcome fear or other obstacles, he has greater self-efficacy. An example of this is self-injecting, which is how most of the current disease-modifying therapies are taken. Nobody likes to give himself or herself a shot, some people are downright terrified of it, and very few of us have experience doing it before we are prescribed one of these medications. However, once a person works through his distaste, fear, and inexperience to successfully inject himself a couple of times, these feelings are diminished in proportion to his sense of accomplishment and his growing self-efficacy. The message here is to make it your goal to succeed once at a new challenge. Then have the goal of succeeding again. If you set small, attainable goals like this, your chances of success go up and you can skirt around much of the stress that comes from looking at the "I-can't-believe-that-I-have-to-do-this-every-day-for-the-rest-of-my-life" big picture.

Observe "peers" succeed. Another influence on self-efficacy is seeing people similar to yourself succeed. Most of us have seen people in pharmaceutical educational materials inject themselves, usually while smiling and sitting in their perfect kitchens. I don't know about you, but I surely wasn't convinced that the process would be as pleasant as it was portrayed. On the other hand, visiting with people in a forum for MS or going to a support group and listening to others talk about their first injections, the difficulties they faced, and how they kept trying (and succeeding) anyway, will do much more to convince you of your ability to do the same thing. In addition to "modeling" the behavior of successfully injecting, these interactions also have the benefit of providing tips and ideas, based on people's real-life experiences and trial and error. Interactions with others with MS in different situations also can be the source of valuable motivation in the form of "pep talks," also known as social persuasion. Remember this source of fortification as you face the different challenges that pop up in your life with MS— others have been there and they can help.

Monitor and adapt your reactions to situations. Our level of self-efficacy is also determined by how we physically and emotionally feel as we tackle challenges and how we interpret these feelings. For instance, say we give ourselves an injection that is particularly painful one day. A person with high self-efficacy might be proud that they persevered despite the pain, whereas a person with low self-efficacy may use the pain as "evidence" that they don't know how to correctly administer a shot, that they *must* be doing something wrong. This can feed into a cycle of positive emotions in the person with high self-efficacy, who will decide that he or she will do better next time, or that a little bit of transient pain is better than the symptoms and relapses the medication is preventing. Our person with low self-efficacy can head into a negative emotional spiral, deciding that they will never get the hang of injecting themselves, eventually leading to the conviction that the medicine probably won't work anyway.

That's all well and good, you might say (if you haven't written all of this off as bogus pop psychology), but how does it break down into action? Albert Bandura, the "father" of the theory of self-efficacy, defines it as "people's beliefs about their **capabilities** to produce designated levels of **performance** that exercise **influence** over events that affect their lives."[2]

For the sake of illustration, **"influence"** translates into "I have a problem, but it can be solved or mitigated." In other words, one must believe that it is not fate alone, nor cosmic forces of any type, determining the course of events. It implies that, despite the magnitude of the obstacle or problem, a solution exists in the world, which brings us to the **"performance"** in the definition. This is the plan of attack and subsequent measures taken that *will* get us to our solution. The third vital component is you. It is not enough to believe that a problem can be solved and have ideas as to how this can be done—you have to be confident that *you* are **capable** of putting the actions into motion and following through until there is some sort of relief or resolution.

Do Your Best

Believe that you will succeed in everything that you are doing, even when you don't. Then try again.

I'll give an example from my own life in the interest of keeping it real and avoiding cheesy "everything-always-turns-out-fine-in-the-end" fabricated examples. When I was a brand-new mom of brand-new twins, things were a blur: I was relieved not to be pregnant anymore, there was a flurry of activity and help, and I was riding the symptom-free wave of a bolus of Solu-Medrol that I had gotten for a severe relapse when the twins were three weeks old. However, as happens in pretty much every situation, eventually excitement died down, novelty wore off, and there I was alone with them. I found myself looking at these tiny infants through eyes bleary with MS fatigue, made worse by new-parent exhaustion. There were honestly many days when I sat, blinking back tears, wondering how in the hell I was supposed to meet all of the needs of those little creatures when I felt like I was barely keeping my grip on the edge of the cliff myself.

I can't say that I had an epiphany or that there was a certain moment that I said to myself, "Now, darn it, it's time to put that good ol' self-efficacy to some use." It was more of a realization that this *had* to work, a squaring of the shoulders and setting the goal, each day, of getting through that day mostly intact. It wasn't pretty—it was bumpy, with lots of weeping on all sides, spit-up covered shirts (mine) worn for days in a row, and naps taken on my knees with my face planted in the ottoman. But we did it. One day, then the next. And, sure enough, each little success made me more confident. I found other moms who told me that I was doing great and gave me tips on maximizing efficiency. I started thinking of my aching back, breasts, head, and C-section scar as signs that I was a mom—a good mom, trying my best. This whole experience made integrating the daily injections of Copaxone into my life, as well as dealing with random MS symptoms, easier—I knew I could cope with pretty much anything, even if it didn't resemble any of my preconceived ideas of what it meant to go through life in a state of cool grace and proud dignity.

Eliminate Self-Limiting Beliefs

You may have heard about the "placebo effect," which is a phenomenon whereby a treatment (even a sugar pill) has a positive effect on a symptom or illness, mostly because the person taking it believes in it. Guess what? It works in the opposite way, too. Called the "nocebo effect," if you believe something is bad, that nothing can make you feel better, that a symptom is only going to get worse, or that there is no way you will feel good enough to leave the house that day, there is a *very* good likelihood that you are going to be right.

Know Your Stuff

The placebo effect is the response your body has to something that has no known physiological benefit. It represents the power of belief.

Repeated thoughts take on a certainty, meaning that if your brain replays the message "I am sick, I can't do it," pretty soon you'll be completely convinced. Likewise, if you allow your mind to dwell on the "Why me?" aspects of MS, you'll never get to the "What next?" parts. Self-limiting beliefs are convictions about yourself that get you stuck, but they can be eliminated with a little effort. First, you have to be able to identify your particular self-limiting beliefs and become aware of the times when they are pushing their way into your thoughts. You then have to create more positive beliefs and actively replace your self-limiting thoughts with these. Although this might sound like common sense or even a little silly, it actually can prove to be difficult, as you may not realize just how ingrained some of these beliefs are and how much you are defined by them.

Here are the steps to eliminating self-limiting beliefs, with some examples:

Make a list. Take 15 to 30 minutes to make a list of every negative or self-limiting thought and belief that you have about yourself or how your MS is making your life difficult. Some examples might include: "I don't have the energy to make change." "The pain is too much." "I am too overwhelmed." "There is nothing I can do about my MS." "I don't have time." "I don't have the resources I need." "I don't understand what is happening in my body." "Why me?" Write one thought per line on a piece of paper. Try to think of as many of these beliefs as you can.

Create a follow-up thought. Next to each thought, you need to create a counterargument to use as a follow-up thought. This statement can often start with a "but," or can simply be another statement about you. For example, if your negative thought was "I don't feel well enough to exercise," your counterargument could be "but it might make me feel better, so it is worth a shot. I can always stop if it makes me feel worse." One thing that I had to work on following my diagnosis was the recording that played in my head, saying, "I can't have fun because my MS hug is too painful." This resulted in me staying home and missing out on things. But one day I thought, "the stupid pain will be there whether I go out or not, so I might as well see if I can have fun and maybe get distracted from it." It worked about two-thirds of the time— I actually had a nice time—and the times when the pain prevented fun were no worse than if I had stayed home anyway. Remember that you don't always have to believe 100% in your counterargument, this is more like ongoing experimentation to uncover areas in which improvement can be made. It helps to write down the counterarguments that you come up with so that you can review your list occasionally.

The Real World

If you can't convince yourself, you'll *never* convince anyone else.

Use the follow-up. Every time you think one of your negative or self-limiting thoughts, always add the follow-up. It might take you some time to catch yourself thinking or saying the negative thoughts, but you will be more aware of them every day. By adding the counterargument, *even if you don't believe it*, you'll be reducing the power of the negative thoughts to influence you. Eventually, they will come less frequently.

Here are some tips for eliminating, or at least reducing, your number of self-limiting beliefs and the power they have over you:

Have faith. This exercise may seem contrived and difficult, but it truly does work. You really can retrain your brain using this technique. It takes some practice and some patience, but it will expand your confidence in yourself.

Make a really good list of your negative and self-limiting beliefs. You may think that you do not have very many of these types of thoughts, but every person has dozens, or even hundreds, of them. Make your list. If you are having trouble thinking of them, pay attention to your thinking as you go through the day—you are sure to find some negative and self-limiting thoughts that are standing in your way.

Recognize that making the counterarguments can be difficult. You may be so convinced of your negative or limiting belief that you can't see any alternative. Don't let yourself off the hook. How would someone you admire deal with the situation? What would your family say about that? What would you like to believe instead? Find a way to counterargue. Your follow-ups can change over time, but don't let one negative belief go by without challenging it.

Do Your Best

Develop a voice inside your head that is always positive and ready to argue with your negative thoughts. You probably already hear the negative voice talking to you loud and clear; it's time to find the positive one.

Have the courage to let go of your limitations. You may have actually grown fond of some of your negative and limiting beliefs, and may have even built parts of your personality around them, which means this exercise will be particularly difficult. Stick with it and try not to be afraid of what happens when you let go for a little while. Remember, you don't have to believe the counterarguments, just try to shake things up a little.

Add the counterargument to your speech as well as your thoughts. If you hear yourself telling someone "I just can't remember things," be sure to follow with a counterargument like, "but I'm going to try using lists to see if that might help." Don't let yourself make negative statements without challenging them.

Present Yourself (And Your MS) to the World on Your Own Terms

We all have lain awake in bed rewinding and replaying situations and conversations that happened earlier that day (or if it was really bad, that week or month), mentally replacing our awkward or goofy or stupid or nonsensical contributions to the interaction with flawless responses that flowed seamlessly as evidence of our amazing intellect and social dexterity. Although we cannot predict when someone is going to spring politics or religion or an esoteric/distasteful/bizarre topic on us, we pretty much know that our MS will be the topic of conversation at some point with certain people.

Too often, those of us with MS cannot communicate what is happening to us, especially if we are caught off-guard or having a bad day. Of course it is difficult—not only does MS affect us on many levels simultaneously, it can also stir up feelings of anxiety, humiliation, and loneliness that are extremely personal and difficult to both talk about and edit at the same time. This may leave the people around us confused and uncertain, but it also takes a big bite out of our confidence when we are unable to express ourselves in a way that makes us proud of ourselves, rather than second-guessing and replaying what we have said to different people.

This is not necessarily about disclosing your MS status to others. Preparing yourself to talk about MS is more about arming you with materials so that you are in control of a potentially awkward situation and can be confident that you will be ready to present the you that you want the world to see.

Write a 30-Second Speech About Your MS

I have a friend who was recently diagnosed with lupus. She is pretty private about her life and really doesn't like to share medical information with many people, although we have in-depth discussions about our respective conditions. Not too long ago, she called me in a sputtering rage. She had just gotten off the phone with a friend with whom she had to cancel some plans, citing "a couple little health problems" as the reason. Her friend didn't merely ask what the problem was, she practically reached through the phone demanding details, saying, "Tell me from the beginning! What is it again? How do you spell it? Did you get a second opinion? Why not?! Tell me everything!" My friend was angry at her, but more upset with herself, because, as she said, "I wanted to stop talking, but I couldn't. I was so flustered and taken off-guard that I was telling this person everything, including details I don't even share with my husband." I've been there before—situations where I end up dismayed that I disclosed such personal details, while also berating myself for letting myself become a social "victim" of someone's whims.

Preparing a speech about your MS may seem like a bizarre exercise, especially if you have been living with multiple sclerosis for awhile. You may be thinking to yourself that everyone pretty much knows how you are doing. But think about it for a moment. If you are like me, your MS takes you on a roller coaster ride most days. I know that I can be caught off-guard by symptoms like fatigue and pain and so swept up in the moment that if I was to tell people about my MS at that very second, they would think that I was completely unable to cope. There are other times that I am truly feeling okay (comparatively) and when I talk about my MS at those times, it comes across as really no big deal, which is also far from accurate.

The Real World

Salesmen are trained with 30-second "elevator pitches" about their product or service, in which they explain a concept and "hook" someone. We need to get our MS "stories" out there just as efficiently and effectively.

There are also certain people to whom I have a more difficult time expressing myself, so I end up doing a poor job of it. Some of these people seem too busy to listen to details, others have their own stories to tell, others I just find downright intimidating (like priests or Parisians), although I would like to communicate with them.

Writing a 30-second "speech" about your MS on a sheet of paper is one way to tackle this predicament. Think about including the following information: what type of MS you have, how severe your symptoms are at the moment and how they are impacting your life, what you are doing to cope with your symptoms, and your attitude toward MS.

Here is my sample:

"As you probably remember, I have relapsing-remitting MS and I have been pretty lucky in that I have not had a relapse for awhile. I am a little frustrated with my symptoms these days, though. My fatigue just makes normal things difficult—I mean, I never loved housework, but now it requires strategic planning to get the dishwasher unloaded in one day. On the other hand, I have started exercising—just 30 minutes on the treadmill—and that seems to give me a little energy boost that buys me a couple of good hours in the morning. I was also pretty happy at my last neurologist appointment when he said that some of my old lesions were shrinking, so that probably explains why I can feel my feet again on good days. Overall, he seemed to think that I was doing well, and I can honestly say that my ups and downs are evening out a little."

Okay, I timed myself on that speech. 40 seconds. Not bad. I couldn't resist adding the line about feeling my feet again. I call an element like that the "Holy shit!" moment, which informs the listener that this MS thing is a pretty big deal and gives them a concrete sensation to relate to that really conveys what I am going through. You can make the decision whether or not to include your own "Holy shit!" moment or not. Try it out—you may find it strangely gratifying.

Make sure that you practice your speech a couple of times. What you are aiming for is not rote memorization, but to capture the right feeling and elements that will convey what you want to get across. For me it is important that certain people know that I am struggling with fatigue, but trying things to help myself. I also want them to not think that I am covering something up, but sharing an appropriate amount of information.

Make It Better

Those of us with MS cannot truly change things about life with this disease until we can articulate our thoughts and feelings about ourselves, our lives, and our multiple sclerosis.

Create more than one 30-second speech if you need to. Clearly, you will have different approaches if you are explaining things to young children in your extended family, to a parent of your child's classmate, or to your cousin. Take some time and think about the tone you want to set when you talk to people about your MS. Maybe you are looking for sympathy, maybe you are simply informing people, maybe you are looking for advice, or maybe you want a little of the "Holy shit!" reaction. You can set the appropriate tone.

You can also take this exercise to the next level by finding ways to educate others about your condition. Maybe you will start with friends or family members. Explain what you know, tell people about MS disease progression, talk about the latest treatments. Make it interesting. Use your communication skills and your life experience to make a difference. Tell your story.

Deal With Some MS FAQs

This exercise is related to the 30-second speech in that you are preparing yourself to respond to questions, rather than getting caught like a deer in the headlights when people ask something that probably seems innocent enough to them, but stirs up a whole bunch of emotions in you.

Do Your Best

You will be asked questions, many of which will seem ignorant or insensitive. Decide ahead of time if you want to deal with these questions with quiet, patient grace, or to firmly educate your audience—it's up to you, as long as you aren't a victim of the moment.

Sit down with some paper and take time to list questions people have asked or could ask about MS. Depending on how long your list is, you may need to choose the questions that are asked most frequently—these are your FAQs. Write an answer for each question. Decide on the tone and emotional quality that you want to respond with. Make your answers as detailed as you like. You may have different answers to the same question, depending on if it is your spouse, mother, child, or a random lady at the grocery store asking it.

Here are some of my FAQs:

- Isn't it hard to work/raise children/whatever when you have MS?
- I saw Montel Williams talk about his MS. You don't feel as bad as he does, do you?
- What do the doctors think is going to happen to you?
- Aren't you taking medicine for your MS? Isn't it helping?
- Why are you so tired all the time?

It really helps me to have thought out the answers to these questions. This preparation has actually saved me in the past from reacting emotionally and either lashing out in pure, blind rage or bursting into tears, when I am sure the person asking the question had absolutely no idea that they were hitting a nerve.

The Bottom Line

Whether you just picked up this book on your way home from the appointment where the neurologist told you that you have MS or you are a veteran MSer, from now on—every day for the rest of your life—you will have a choice as to how you will live that day as a person with MS.

I am not Pollyannaish about having MS. I have it too, and I know that some things are simply out of our control. I do not know how fatigued I will feel, or whether I will be able to carry on a coherent conversation when it is most crucial. I do not know which activities I will be able to do with my family, later this afternoon, next month, two years from now. I cannot tell you that I will not be scared at times or not get so angry that I snap at those whom I love for no reason besides that they are there when I need a target.

But I can tell you this—I will not give in to this disease, as corny and tiresome as that may sound. I will cling to the confidence that I can do something. Then I will do it—or at least do the best I can. It might not be what I had pictured myself doing, or hoped that I could do, but I will keep going, will keep doing.

2

Be an MS Expert

You *Must* Understand Your MS

The day after I got my initial diagnosis of multiple sclerosis, July 9, 2004, I left to go to a scientific conference in Thailand. I had a bottle containing pills of small daily doses of oral prednisone and a book about MS that had been written in 1992 that I'd found in a bookstore on my way home from my doctor's appointment. I won't go into detail about the horror of being in a completely unfamiliar environment while taking an anxiety-inducing drug that should have never been prescribed in the first place. The information that I had was so outdated that the best advice it could offer was for me to rest, avoid stress, and plan to make my life easier for my imminent disability. I had also been told—incorrectly—by the neurologist who diagnosed me that heat could bring on a relapse, so I spent the majority of my trip making frantic, fear-filled dashes between air-conditioned venues, rather than enjoying any aspect of Bangkok. Needless to say, I could have had a much more pleasant trip, and started out my life as a person living with MS in a more positive way, if I had just been armed with the correct information.

Know Your Stuff

You *must* understand your illness, your symptoms, and your medications if you are going to be in control of your life. There is no other choice.

In the world of public health, there is much discussion of a concept called "health literacy." Health literacy is defined in *Healthy People 2010* as: "The degree to which individuals have the capacity to obtain, process, and understand basic health information and services needed to make appropriate health decisions."[1] In most cases, when a deficit of health literacy is discussed, it is in reference to low-literate people or people incapable of making decisions, which ultimately translates into poorly-monitored and untreated diabetes, high blood pressure, or cardiac problems. Many people in these situations are afraid to ask questions, do not fully understand their diagnoses, or are overwhelmed by prescribed treatment regimens or medication side effects, all of which leads to reduced adherence and worsening health.

Know Your Stuff

Health literacy is the capacity of a person to process the health information necessary to make the decision that is best for them. For those of us with MS to be truly health literate, we will pull information from neurology, psychology, clinical trial research, immunology, and sometimes even fields like urology and acupuncture. You need to become your own expert; no one else can do it for you.

As people with MS, the degree of health literacy that we need to attain in order to meet the definition above goes far beyond being functionally literate and understanding the logistics involved with keeping appointments with a physician. MS is a very complicated disease—a vast jumble of over eighty possible symptoms stirred in with a big mess of confusing treatment options. It is likely that if you visited several neurologists, each one would have a different recommendation, or they might just toss the options back in your lap for you to choose from. Under these circumstances, the health literacy that is required to "make appropriate health decisions" is overwhelming, even considered by many people with MS to be out of reach. So they give up.

Not comprehending the basic principles of MS makes every symptom a surprise, and decisions get scarier. Think for a moment—what possibilities could you be missing out on because of a deficiency of understanding about your own illness? Developing a specific skill set around finding the answers that you need in order to discuss things with your doctor, calm your nerves, or know what to expect, is essential. An often-overlooked aspect of living with MS is that each person needs to intimately understand his or her *own* MS, to be able to discuss his or her status with doctors, to know what effects his or her medications are having, and to sense where he or she is in terms of well-being and disease progression. How a person with MS "feels" is a complicated combination of symptoms, both intermittent and constant, side effects from medications, and how he or she reacts to and copes with these physical states.

Quick and Dirty MS Facts

Before we even get started on this section, I have to give a disclaimer on the word "facts" in the section header. There are many things about MS that are known to be true (beyond a reasonable doubt, until proven otherwise); however, there are many more aspects of this disease that escape being pinned down and earning the title of "fact." We don't know what causes MS, we don't know how to cure MS, we cannot always predict the prognosis of individual people with MS, we don't know when the symptoms of a relapse will completely resolve or if there will be residual damage, and we can't be sure that a given treatment is going to work for an individual. Hell, there are even doctors that argue that certain symptoms that many of us experience, such as pain, are in no way connected with MS.

So that leaves us with some stuff that we are pretty sure of, large gaps in knowledge, and a whole bunch of educated guesses. I'm going to do my best to present you with the latest research on the basic aspects of MS, and to also encourage you to stay curious, question everything, keep looking for information, and remain flexible in your thinking about this disease. If a specific concept interests you, or you have the inevitable question or doubt about something, do research— some guidelines are provided later in this chapter. You will find that even a very narrow question opens up a Pandora's box of different opinions from "experts," as well as from people living with MS. Don't get discouraged—question what is written here, question your doctor, question everything until you feel comfortable with the answer.

What is MS?

Let's start with what MS is—a chronic disease of the central nervous system, probably autoimmune in nature. "**Chronic**" means that MS is not curable, period. Even though there are promising treatments that seem to be slowing down the progression of MS in some cases, as well as people making claims about diet, alternative therapies, and other "cures," to date, there is no cure for MS. Chronic also implies that the disease hangs out for a long time, as opposed to an acute illness, which does its stuff fast and is either cured, resolves on its own, or kills you quickly. As a disease of the **central nervous system**, MS affects the brain and spinal cord (and optic nerves). Although the exact mechanism has not been pinned down, it is pretty clear that MS is an **autoimmune** disease, which means that for some reason, the body's own immune system is attacking the myelin surrounding your nerves. Myelin is the soft, white, fatty sheath that surrounds the nerve structures and helps conduct signals.

MS causes symptoms in three ways—by creating inflammation, scars, and atrophy. These things happen with different frequency or order in the different types of MS. **Inflammation** occurs when the attack is happening—certain immune cells start going after the myelin, and this process signals other cells to the area, causing swelling and irritation (think of a mosquito bite, but on your brain, as nasty as that might sound). This acute reaction is the cause of relapses, because the inflamed area is bigger than the actual "injury" to the myelin, but the swelling impedes electrical signals from traveling efficiently down the nerves. Eventually—more specifically, after four to six weeks when untreated or more quickly following a dose of corticosteroids—the inflammation recedes and some degree of healing (remyelination) occurs. This remyelination is usually imperfect, leaving a **scar** in the form of a lesion, which often causes residual symptoms. The third way that MS results in symptoms is through atrophy. **Atrophy** refers to loss of brain and spinal cord tissue and occurs when the entire nerve structure (myelin, as well as the axons that it surrounds) has been destroyed. This loss can result in disseminated atrophy, a generalized shrinkage of the spinal cord and brain, as well as black holes, which are localized areas where the brain tissue is destroyed.

Know Your Stuff

Corticosteroids suppress the immune system, in turn reducing the inflammation that is causing symptoms. A hefty dose of corticosteroids can shorten the duration and severity of relapses in many cases.

What are the Types of MS?

At present, there are four types of MS: relapsing-remitting, secondary-progressive, primary-progressive, and progressive-relapsing. Though this may seem simple enough, there is some controversy and confusion around classifying the different presentations of MS in this way. Many experts believe that the different types of multiple sclerosis may actually represent different diseases because of how they present clinically and their dissimilar appearances on MRI scans. You may also hear the four types referred to as different "stages" or "phases" of MS, but these are misleading (and incorrect) terms, because one type does not necessarily lead to another.

Too often, the topic of multiple sclerosis is treated as relapsing-remitting MS (RRMS) only. Although most people start out diagnosed with RRMS, there are many people that do not; instead they are diagnosed with progressive MS from the beginning. Many who start out with an RRMS diagnosis later get reclassified as having secondary progressive MS. And let's not forget our friends who get the "double-whammy" of relapsing-progressive MS, the form in which you progress and have relapses, but do not experience remission. Each of these types has specific characteristics and challenges. We'll go over each type below.

Relapsing-Remitting MS

The majority (about 85%) of people with MS receive an initial diagnosis of relapsing-remitting MS. This type of MS is characterized by definite periods of relapses, then a "remitting" of symptoms. This does not necessarily mean that the symptoms disappear entirely; people either return to the level of disability where they were before the relapse or are left with some residual damage from the relapse. For example, a person may walk again after a relapse during which they were unable to walk, but they might have a limp. In my case, I lost sight completely in one eye during a bout of optic neuritis, which was restored with a course of Solu-Medrol, but colors seen with that eye are still dim and faded. It should also be noted that disability often continues to progress in RRMS even without acute relapses, although it might be slow and subtle.

Know Your Stuff

Solu-Medrol is the most common steroid given to shorten an MS relapse. Solu-Medrol is given through an IV and can cause side effects like anxiety and sleep problems. I have had fairly severe symptoms completely disappear during the course of my first two-hour infusion. On the other hand, I also suffered from extreme anxiety during the five days of my treatment course, which was helped only by a small dose of Ativan.

Secondary-Progressive MS

Secondary-progressive MS (SPMS) starts out as relapsing-remitting MS, meaning that people are usually first diagnosed with RRMS, and then their diagnosis changes, as their MS becomes more progressive in nature. It is possible that some people receive an initial diagnosis of SPMS because the relapses that they had in the past went undiagnosed as MS.

Know Your Stuff

Disease-modifying therapies are medications that are taken to slow the progression of MS. These therapies do not treat symptoms nor cure MS.

Before disease-modifying therapies became widely available, 80 to 90% of people with RRMS would eventually develop SPMS within 25 years (50% within 10 years). It is now unclear what effect these medications will have on MS progression, but it is assumed and hoped that this proportion will be much lower and that people taking these therapies will be slower to develop SPMS.

Although it is difficult to predict with certainty which people living with RRMS will go on to develop SPMS, there are some factors that make progression more likely, but NOT certain. These factors are: male gender, later age (older than 40) at diagnosis with RRMS, and living with MS for 5 to 20 years. To me, the last two factors are artifactual, meaning that people living with RRMS for longer before diagnosis will probably be older, and the longer you live with RRMS, the greater the chance that it will progress.

There are some signs that RRMS is progressing into SPMS. The CRAB (Copaxone, Rebif, Avonex, Betaseron) drugs and Tysabri stop working as well, meaning that the person will have increased disability, despite good adherence. Relapses become more severe, they are characterized by multiple symptoms and reduced or no response to Solu-Medrol, and they begin to leave more residual symptoms or disability in their wake. When disability, measured by the Expanded Disability Status Scale (EDSS), reaches a level of 4 to 5.5 (indicated by the inability to walk more than 500 meters without resting), this is an indication that the person will probably develop SPMS within a short time. The doctor will find more abnormal signs during the neurological exams, indicating that the brain can no longer compensate for the demyelination. Along the same lines, people who develop SPMS tend to exhibit more cognitive disturbances, again likely due to the greater degree of atrophy in the brain. MRI scans show more damage, in the form of a greater lesion burden (total number of lesions) and more atrophy. Interestingly, the number of active, gadolinium-enhancing lesions decreases in the later stages of RRMS, as the disease is likely becoming more degenerative than inflammatory.

Know Your Stuff

Gadolinium is used during an MRI. It is a fluid put into your body that "lights up" areas of your brain and spinal cord that are actively inflamed.

I am going to take this opportunity to make a very important point: MS progression is not anyone's fault. I was angered beyond words to read in a book for newly diagnosed people that they should *set a goal* of having inactive MS (defined by that author as no relapses for five years). This author implied that "caring for yourself diligently" and "treating your MS actively" during the first year following diagnosis can help you achieve this objective. Sure, for *some* people the current medications might help reduce the number of relapses—if they can obtain the drugs, if they have the "right" kind of MS (RRMS), if they can tolerate the drugs, if they don't produce neutralizing antibodies, if their MS decides to cooperate, if the stars line up in their favor. For some people, these drugs don't click with them or with their MS. Asserting that anything that we do or don't do can stop the progression of our MS inevitably sets some of us up to be failures in the business of living with MS.

Primary-Progressive MS

About 15% of people are initially diagnosed with primary-progressive MS (PPMS), a form of the disease in which there are no relapses, but a steady course of progression. This can be so subtle at first that it may take several years to reach diagnosis. Most people (about 85%) who are eventually diagnosed with PPMS begin noticing that they are having problems walking, which gradually get worse; however, the first symptoms of about 10% of people with PPMS are slowly worsening tremor and problems with balance. Though rare, the following symptoms can also be signs of PPMS in about 3 to 5% of people: brainstem syndrome (difficulties with swallowing, hoarseness, dizziness, nausea, and vomiting); rapid involuntary movements of the eyes; progressively worsening vision; and cognitive dysfunction.

The MRI scans of the brains of people with PPMS show few lesions and often no gadolinium-enhancing lesions, which makes diagnosis extra challenging. However, an MRI scan of the spine will often show atrophy, which is a result of axon and oligodenrocyte cell loss. Some experts think that PPMS is a different disease from RRMS because PPMS seems primarily degenerative in nature and RRMS is characterized more by inflammation.

Even well-trained neurologists often miss a diagnosis of PPMS because they are looking for gadolinium-enhancing lesions and acute and defined relapses and remission periods. As people with MS, we must do our part to include those with other forms of MS, regardless of type, in our discussions, and also educate people that other types of MS exist. We can only benefit from the inclusion of all—learning from each other, supporting each another, and keeping others with different types of MS in mind as we advocate for ourselves.

Progressive-Relapsing MS

Although estimates vary from 5 to 10% of people with MS receiving a diagnosis of progressive-relapsing multiple sclerosis (PPMS), it is unquestionably the most rare type. It usually starts out diagnosed as primary-progressive MS, with the disease following a steady course of progression; however, at some point, the person also experiences relapses of acute symptoms, at which point the diagnosis will be changed to progressive-relapsing MS. This course of PRMS is the opposite scenario from SPMS, in which relapses come first (RRMS), followed by steady progression and worsening disability.

The Real World

Us folks with MS have to stick together. Certainly the experience of MS differs depending on MS type and severity, but we still have a lot in common. We all have MS and it can be terrible in different ways, but we can help each other.

What Causes MS?

This is perhaps the biggest "I don't know" aspect of MS. Not only do I not know what causes MS, neither does anyone else. However, with great regularity, readers of my Web site write to me to me, saying, "My MS was caused by surgery (mercury fillings, an accident, aspartame, stress, a vaccine...)."

Know Your Stuff

Many scientists point to vitamin D as one element leading to the development of MS in people. One theory is that people with MS have a genetic deficiency around metabolizing vitamin D, which may lead to an autoimmune response.

I'm not going to argue that any of these things do or do not contribute to MS. Nonetheless, I can state pretty boldly that there is not one single thing that directly causes MS. Rather, there is a combination of things at work, including genetics, geography, and/or exposure to infections. It might go something like this: (1) we have a genetic vulnerability in our DNA, which in turn (2) makes our bodies inefficient at metabolizing vitamin D, in addition to which (3) we may not have gotten enough exposure to the sun (maybe because of geography—far from the equator—or because we just did not go outside much) to allow us to make enough vitamin D to compensate for the problem, then (4) we get an infection (maybe mononucleosis) that tweaks our immune system the wrong way, maybe even because of the effects of vitamin D deficiency on certain parts of the immune system. This sequence of events, of course, is all theoretical, but it does encompass much of the thinking about the factors that combine to make MS.

Know Your Stuff

Another factor at play in MS may be the Epstein-Barr virus (which causes mononucleosis). It may be that people with MS have a genetic predisposition to "overreact" to the very common Epstein-Barr virus, resulting in MS several years after infection.

Of course, any of the above factors can also be directly or indirectly influenced by other "ingredients" thrown into the recipe. For instance, people who begin smoking early in life, or who smoke several packs a day, are much more likely to get MS than non-smokers. This could be the result of smoking reducing vitamin D levels or directly messing with the immune system (or some entirely different factor). Stress has also been shown to contribute to MS risk, possibly because of the effect of fluctuations in cortisol levels on the immune system.

How Common is MS and Who Gets It?

The best estimate is that 2.5 million people in the world have MS.

It appears that certain genetic combinations increase the likelihood of a person to develop MS, however, the increase in risk is not high enough to call MS a "genetic disease." Instead, it seems that genes are one factor, among many, that determine a person's risk for MS. There was a big hullabaloo in 2007 when scientists discovered two genes linked to MS, which led some to believe that having these genes "caused" MS in the same way that cystic fibrosis is a genetic disease. Instead of a direct causal link, the "MS genes" increase susceptibility to MS, but other factors are at play. It turns out that people with these genes are 20 to 30% more likely to have MS. To translate into real numbers, if the overall risk of MS in the United States is 1 in 1,000, and you have these genes, your risk becomes 1 in 770.

Having a relative with MS increases your chances of developing MS. More specifically, the likelihood of having MS is approximately:

- 1 in 1,000 if you have no relatives with MS

- 1 in 100 if you have a second-degree relative (grandparent, aunt, uncle, etc.) with MS

- 1 in 40 if you have a parent or sibling with MS

- 1 in 4 if your identical twin has MS

Most MS is diagnosed between the ages of 20 and 50, though both childhood and late-onset MS occur. In most parts of the world, women are 2 to 3 times more likely than men to be diagnosed with MS.

MS occurs more frequently in regions that are farther from the equator (above 40 degrees latitude), with the highest prevalence per 100,000 in Canada (240), Hungary (176), and the United Kingdom (164)—the United States is up there with a prevalence of 135 per 100,000 population. MS occurs more often in people of northern European descent, but other ethnicities may also have MS. If a person migrates from a high-risk region to a low-risk region before the age of fifteen, they take on the lower risk. Researchers think that sex hormones and geography, again probably linked to exposure to sunlight and the resulting vitamin D production, may somehow interact to increase MS risk.

The Real World

When people ask how you "got MS," often what they are really asking is "could this happen to me too?" Prepare for this question when you tell someone about MS, and try not to let it make you too angry or hurt your feelings.

If you are interested to see how common MS is in different countries, check out the Atlas of MS database (www.atlasofms.org). This is a fascinating compilation of information about the global multiple sclerosis situation, which includes not only the prevalence of MS in different countries, but also data such as male/female ratio, mean age of onset, and the availability of services and treatment for people living with MS. Every time I come here with a specific question, I get drawn in to the data and find myself rubbing my eyes and blinking much later, head swimming with facts like "there are forty people in Ethiopia living with MS" or "the number of Afghani men and women with MS is the same, whereas in Mongolia, women are seven times more likely to be diagnosed with MS."[2]

How is MS Diagnosed and How is It Monitored Once a Diagnosis is Made?

In times past, MS was diagnosed using the "hot bath test." The person exhibiting suspicious symptoms would be placed in a hot bath and observed by the physician. If the symptoms worsened or new ones appeared, a diagnosis of MS was made. Simple enough.

Although things are improving on the diagnostics front, many cases of MS still evade diagnosis. There are several reasons for this, including: more than eighty symptoms are linked to MS and each person develops symptoms differently; many of the symptoms mimic problems that occur with other diseases; there is no blood test for MS; symptoms usually come and go; and many symptoms are vague and hard to quantify, such as fatigue, sexual dysfunction, depression, and cognitive difficulties. Often these symptoms get attributed to stress by general practitioners and people may never have an MRI scan performed or get referred to a neurologist.

Don't Panic

Remember that your MS doesn't know when the doctor diagnosed you. For those of us living with multiple sclerosis, diagnosis is a defining event, but the MS has probably been part of your life for years or even decades before you were diagnosed. Keep that in mind to get some perspective on how it will impact your life. At the moment of diagnosis, MS has already been part of your past—the difference is that now you know that it is part of your future, too.

In my case, the very competent neurologist that finally gave me my diagnosis of "definitive MS" estimated that I had MS for at least fifteen years before my diagnosis, based on things he saw on an MRI. Sure enough, I could think back that many years to a series of tremors, sensory symptoms, and cognitive clues, which took me to many doctors (including some neurologists), but never resulted in a diagnosis.

The widespread use of MRIs is improving the speed and accuracy of diagnosis of MS for some, but many cases still evade diagnosis, especially if the findings on the MRI are difficult to interpret or atypical. Let's have a look at the tools the doctor uses to determine MS status, which include: MRI scans, medical history, neurological exams, evoked potential testing, and lumbar punctures. The first three are also the main ways to monitor MS progression and response to treatment, so they will be repeated—usually on an annual basis or when a relapse is suspected—whereas evoked potentials and lumbar punctures are usually only done once, unless circumstances warrant repeating them.

Magnetic Resonance Imaging (MRI) Scan

MRI scanners use magnetic waves to produce hundreds of cross-section images of the brain and spinal cord (often just the cervical, or neck, area of the spine is imaged). A special contrast material (gadolinium) is usually injected for the scan when MS is suspected because it reacts to areas of inflammation and will "light up" when it hits an active lesion, indicating that demyelination is occurring. An MRI is considered the best test for diagnosing MS because abnormal lesions appear on MRIs in over 95% of people with MS; however, 5% of people with MS do not have abnormalities that can be detected on an MRI (producing a false negative), and some age-related damage looks like MS lesions (producing a false positive). In addition, the MRI images of the brains of people with PPMS often show few (if any) lesions and no gadolinium-enhancing lesions. In these cases, however, an MRI scan of the spine will often show a substantial amount of atrophy, which is a result of axon and oligodenrocyte cell loss and injury. The MRI results that may indicate MS are: active (gadolinium-enhancing) lesions, T2-weighted lesions ("black holes" of localized atrophy), and generalized atrophy (areas where the brain has lost volume).

Know Your Stuff

An axon is the "tail" of a neuron that conducts electrical signals away from the nerve and is covered in myelin. An oligodenrocyte is a cell in the brain that can replace myelin. A T2-weighted lesion is a "scar" that shows evidence of MS disease on an MRI image.

MRI scans are used to monitor the disease progression of MS. Many neurologists, like mine, like to see an annual MRI, especially if the person is currently taking a disease-modifying therapy. Other doctors take a more "as needed" approach, requesting an MRI when a relapse is suspected or as a baseline measure before a new therapy is started.

Medical History

For most of us, the whole reason that we eventually make it to a neurologist's (or other doctor's) office to possibly be diagnosed with MS is that we noticed some symptoms that were new, weird, disabling, and/or troubling. Very few of these symptoms, aside from walking speed and visual acuity, can be measured by a doctor. Therefore, our docs completely rely on us to give them critical information. The doctor will ask about current and past symptoms, including questions such as: When did the symptom start? How long did it last? Precisely where is the sensation or loss of function is located? How intense is the symptom, and is it interfering with daily life? Is it constant, or does it come and go? Does anything make it better or worse? It helps to be as accurate and complete as possible in discussing any symptom that you think is relevant. (See Chapter 3, section "How to talk to your doctor about your symptoms" for ideas.) Make a list of all symptoms that you have experienced, even if other doctors told you nothing was wrong, or attributed it to something else.

Do Your Best

Become your own "medical detective" by meticulously recording your medical history, symptoms, and any contributing factors (like stress or poor sleep). Quality of life with MS relies heavily on symptom management, and you may miss opportunities for improvement if you are not paying attention.

You will also need to bring all other medical information along, including which prescription drugs you are taking, any medical test results you may have, and other doctors' findings. You will probably also be asked several questions about the medical history of relatives and drug and alcohol use, as well as other health issues that you may have had in the past.

Of course, in-depth discussions of symptoms since the last visit, any side effects experienced from medications, and any changes in medications or other health conditions are a vital part of monitoring MS and will be repeated during every visit.

Neurologic Exam

To me, this is the most interesting part of the diagnostic process. I love it because the only "tools" that the doctor uses are her hands, an eye chart, a penlight, an ophthalmoscope (small hand-held instrument to look in your eye), a rubber reflex hammer, a vibrating tuning fork, and a broken cotton swab. Using these "primitive" instruments, the doc observes different reactions that you have to stimuli and asks you questions about sensations you feel. She will also have you do things like squeeze her hands, follow a moving penlight with your eyes, and walk on your tiptoes and heels. These tests do not hurt and are very interesting, especially once you know what the doc is looking for. The entire test will probably last about 15 minutes, but may take as long as 2 hours.

Neurological "signs" are impairments or alterations in normal responses that doctors can use to help with diagnosis. They usually do not cause symptoms, but can be observed and measured (an example is Romberg's sign, which is present if you sway when you stand with your arms stretched in front of you and close your eyes). What is really neat is that the doc will know which areas of the nervous system are damaged simply by observing these signs. The doctor will be testing for signs involving the following: functioning of the cranial nerves (these control the senses, as well as how you talk and swallow); coordination; strength; reflexes; and sensation. Whether you realize it or not, the doctor is also carefully observing you to see if you exhibit any signs of depression and listening carefully to your speech patterns for possible speech dysfunction, as both are symptoms of MS.

One thing your doc is doing is placing you (either formally or just in her mind) on the Expanded Disability Status Scale (EDSS), a rating system that is frequently used for classifying and standardizing the condition of people with MS. Although most neurologists do not formally use EDSS scores to monitor their patients, my neurologist told me that he watched approximate disability scores to determine when to take action, such as Solu-Medrol treatment, or whether physical therapy was warranted. Your EDSS can improve, based on successful treatment or if symptoms resolve on their own.

Take Charge

Make each test an opportunity to learn about MS and your body. Learn the details of what the results mean. Be curious about your MS.

Evoked Potential Testing

The three evoked potential tests used in diagnosing multiple sclerosis are visual evoked potentials or responses (VER), somatosensory evoked potentials (SSEP), and brainstem auditory evoked potentials (BAEP). For all of the tests, electrodes are applied to the scalp with some sort of conducting gel. The tests take 30 to 60 minutes each. The stimulations are different for each test. In the VER, the eyes are stimulated by looking at a computer screen that is flashing checkerboard patterns of differing sizes or a strobe-type light while one eye is covered. During the BAEP test, the hearing is stimulated by listening to test tones, beeps or clicks through headphones, usually in a dark room. The SSEP involves the nerves of the arms and legs being stimulated by electrical pulses delivered through electrodes stuck onto the skin, usually at the wrist or knee (but occasionally near an ankle or elbow), which feel like small electric shocks.

An "abnormal" result basically means that the signal took longer to reach the brain or that it was less intense that it normally would be in a person with healthy nerves. VER is the most useful of the evoked potential tests in helping to diagnose MS (85% of people with MS have abnormal results), especially for things like progressive MS that do not show up very well on MRI scans, or to confirm that there is damage that might not show up as a symptom.

Make It Better

Choose your post-test reward. Mine is ice cream. Okay, maybe a new pair of shoes *and* ice cream.

Lumbar Puncture

Also called a spinal tap, this test involves withdrawing a small amount of cerebrospinal fluid from your spinal column with a needle inserted between your vertebrae and testing the fluid in a lab. You may not need to get a lumbar puncture if the results from your MRI, neurological exam, and symptom history point pretty clearly to MS. However, lumbar puncture results can be useful for ruling out other things if there is still a question about diagnosis. A lumbar puncture can also be quite useful (or necessary) for aiding in the diagnosis of PPMS, because MRI results can be difficult to interpret or subtle in progressive forms of MS.

A "positive result" is the presence of oligoclonal bands (an elevated number of certain antibodies), which is an indicator of increased immune activity in the spinal fluid. This test is positive in up to 90% of people with MS, but a positive result could indicate another disease or disorder.

When I talk about lumbar punctures, I am compelled to point out that they can be done using an X-ray technique known as fluoroscopy, which helps the doctor or technician guide the needle, making the procedure faster and less stressful to the person getting "tapped" (and probably to the person doing the procedure, as well). Many residents, interns and less experienced doctors are anxious to perform lumbar punctures without fluoroscopy in order to practice or because they do not have convenient access to the fluoroscopy equipment. Do not hesitate to insist on a fluoroscopy-guided lumbar puncture, even if you have to wait or get referred to another facility for the test. An experienced technician using fluoroscopy has a much greater chance of performing a smooth and quick lumbar puncture.

Blood Tests

Although there is not a blood test for MS, usually a series of blood tests will be run to rule out other things that could cause similar symptoms, such as Lyme disease, HIV, some rare genetic disorders, and a group of diseases known as collagen-vascular diseases (these include lupus, rheumatoid arthritis, scleroderma, and others).

Diagnostic Criteria

Some of you may currently be "in limbo" with your MS diagnosis, meaning that you have not received a positive diagnosis. You could have had one attack of characteristic MS symptoms and lesions that showed up on an MRI, called a clinically isolated syndrome (CIS), but nothing since then. Or, you could have all the symptoms of MS, but MRI evidence is just not there to warrant a definitive diagnosis. Further confusing the issue, I have spoken to several people that actually had the "wrong" type of MRI done for diagnosis. (For an accurate test, make sure that gadolinium is used during your scan and that your cervical spine is included in the series).

Getting an MS diagnosis is a multi-step process. Because multiple sclerosis means multiple areas of damage ("sclerosis" literally means "scarring" or "hardening"), there used to be two basic rules for diagnosing MS:

- The person must have had at least two attacks (episodes where MS symptoms were present), separated by at least one month, and

- There must be more than one lesion on the brain or spinal cord.

This would mean that after only one clinical attack (CIS), the person would have to wait for more symptoms to know if they had MS; however, now MRI results can be used to confirm symptoms after one attack, according to the McDonald criteria, a set of standards published in 2001 (and revised in 2005), that incorporate the use of MRI scans.

Basically, these criteria state that in the case of only one attack, MS can be confirmed by:

- Dissemination in space by two or more MRI lesions consistent with MS, and

- Dissemination in time by 2nd clinical attack or MRI lesions.[3, 4]

There is one very important change in the revised criteria: "dissemination in time by MRI" means that if a person only has one attack and there is at least one lesion on an MRI, a second scan can be performed three months later. If a new lesion appears, this can be used to diagnose MS without waiting for a second clinical relapse.

The Real World

It's not just *you* being diagnosed, it's somebody's daughter, husband, mom, or best friend. Don't forget that your diagnosis impacts other people, too.

Diagnostic Categories

You may also fall into the limbo of having "possible" or "probable" MS. Yes, to complicate things even further, there are four different diagnostic categories of MS. Let's start with the easy ones. "Negative" means negative and you don't have MS (you probably aren't reading this book, either). The doctor can only say this when another definite diagnosis is made that can account for your symptoms. "Definite MS" is also pretty straightforward—your case fits the diagnostic criteria above.

"Possible MS" means you may have an attack of symptoms that look like MS, but your tests (MRIs, evoked potentials, and lumbar puncture) are normal. No other diagnosis has been confirmed that accounts for the symptoms. "Probable MS" is also pretty fuzzy, and many people find themselves here. You may have symptoms that look like MS and have had two separate episodes separated by at least a month, but normal findings on an MRI. You could also have an MRI that showed only one lesion in your brain or spine. In this case, your doctor will probably recommend repeating the MRI after a certain period of time (for instance, 3 months) to see if any other lesions appear. Depending on how certain your doctor is that you really do have MS (or that you are headed that way), he may recommend that you consider starting a disease-modifying therapy.

What is a Relapse?

When a person is first diagnosed with one of the relapsing forms of MS, the tendency is often to assume that every twinge or bad day is an indication that a relapse is right around the corner. The definition of a relapse is: "A clinically significant event (meaning that it has outward signs and/or symptoms) caused by an active lesion on your brain, spinal cord or optic nerves. It is either a worsening of symptoms that you already have, or the appearance of new symptoms. Relapses are also referred to as 'exacerbations,' 'attacks' or 'flares.'"[5] While this information is accurate, it tells us nothing about ourselves and often confirms our fears until we begin to learn more about how *our* MS behaves.

Know Your Stuff

A relapse is the outward manifestation of an active lesion in your brain or spinal cord, resulting in new symptoms or the noticeable worsening of existing symptoms. Residual symptoms are left over from a prior relapse, which can get worse depending on things like stress, heat, and infection.

Most of us have symptoms that are "new" or "worsening" pretty frequently, so how does anyone know whether or not they are having a relapse? Clearly, some relapses are obvious—when I lost vision in my left eye, I astutely identified that as a relapse. The only way to *really* know whether you are having a relapse is to have an MRI with gadolinium (contrast material that is injected during the MRI scan). Gadolinium is drawn to areas of inflammation and "lights up" when a lesion is "active," indicating that demyelination is currently occurring and you are having a true relapse, rather than feeling symptoms caused by older lesions.

Because you probably don't have an MRI scanner at home, there are some questions that you can ask yourself to determine whether this is just "one of those days" or if you need to go see your doctor:

You can suspect a relapse if you answer "yes" to the following questions:

- Am I experiencing new symptoms or worsening of existing symptoms?

- Has this worsening happened over the course of 24 hours to a couple of days?

- Have these symptoms lasted more than 24 hours?

- Has it been at least a month since my last relapse? (In other words, have current symptoms been non-existent or stable for at least 30 days before they appeared or got worse?)

- Am I free of fever or infection?

Make It Better

Train the people you live with to spot symptoms. They may notice some things that are "off" before you do, and be able to cue you to slow down or make a plan.

These will help you to see if you meet the official international definition of a relapse, which is "a period in which a person with MS experiences an acute worsening of function that lasts for at least 24 hours, usually lasting for several days or weeks, followed by an improvement that lasts for at least one month."[6] The duration of most relapses can be significantly reduced using a course of high-dose corticosteroids, usually Solu-Medrol, which quickly reduces the inflammation and the most severe symptoms. Doctors decide to treat a relapse based on how much the symptoms interfere with daily activities or how much discomfort or distress they are causing. The Solu-Medrol is usually given intravenously for 3 to 7 days, 500 to 1,000 mg each day. The most widely-used regimen is 1,000 mg per day for 5 days.

Other Types of MS

Pediatric MS

It is estimated that up to 5% of people with MS have symptoms before they are 16 years old and less than 1% before they are 10 years old. It happens almost three times more often in girls than boys. Diagnosis of MS in children is very difficult and often gets missed for a long time because doctors do not expect to see it and have little experience with it. There are also many other childhood diseases and disorders with the same symptoms as MS that get considered first.

RRMS is the initial form of MS in 97 to 99% of children, and they tend to have the same symptoms as adults, although they are more likely to have optic neuritis, an isolated brainstem syndrome, or encephalitic symptoms (seizures, vomiting, or headaches). MS seems to progress more slowly in children, however, people diagnosed with pediatric MS usually have greater accumulated disability at the same age as people who were diagnosed as adults, due to the sheer amount of time that they have been living with the disease.

Benign MS

Benign MS describes a type of relapsing-remitting multiple sclerosis in which a few mild relapses, usually producing sensory symptoms, occur and then go away, leaving very little (or no) residual damage or disability. It is estimated that 10 to 20% of people with MS have benign MS, but it is impossible to predict who will follow this course. It is also estimated that half (or more) of these people will eventually have MS progression and no longer have benign MS.

There is debate on the topic of exactly how to define benign MS, but some researchers propose a definition of benign MS as applying to the situation of people who have had MS for at least 10 years and who have an Expanded Disability Status Scale (EDSS) score of 2.0 or less. Many neurologists and researchers do not use the term "benign MS," as there is not consensus about the definition and it is hard to estimate numbers of people that could be classified as having it.

Acute Variants of MS

On the opposite end of the spectrum from benign MS are a couple of very rare forms of multiple sclerosis. Marburg type (also known as malignant multiple sclerosis) and Balò's concentric sclerosis are very aggressive forms of the disease. Progression to extreme disability, including blindness and paraplegia, is usually rapid, typically occurring within 2 to 4 weeks from the onset of symptoms. It is usually lethal within a short time period; death is caused by the destruction of vital brainstem structures. However, there are rare cases of people living years after their first bout with this disease.

Clearly, there is so much to know about MS, as well as so many things that remain unknown, that it is difficult for anyone to have a comprehensive understanding of the whole multiple sclerosis universe. Not only is it difficult, for those of us living with MS it is unnecessary— we need to know the specifics of *our* disease and symptoms. One way to get a handle on the information pertinent to our situation is to compile our own "MS encyclopedia."

Create (and Become) an MS Encyclopedia

Once I was hiking with a friend in a park just outside of New York City. We had just negotiated our way down a very steep rocky slope, which scared the hell out of me. Upon my safe descent the bottom, I was bubbly with proud excitement and adrenaline when a dog barked. I turned to see where the dog was and promptly fell on perfectly flat terrain, managing to land on the only sharp rock in the immediate area, which gouged a hole into my knee. The wound bled a little and hurt terribly, but mostly just oozed blood on the ride back to Manhattan.

I went through the usual ER rigmarole—papers, tetanus shot, X-rays—until the teenage-appearing intern showed up. He was muttering something to the nurse about stitches and antibiotics when I took the opportunity to crow, "My knee is leaking synovial fluid." I was so excited to use my fancy new word, which I had learned in the lab where I was working; to me, "synovial fluid" (which is the fluid that lubricates joints) was the kind of term that indicated that I was "in the know" around medical stuff. When he asked me how I knew that, I said, "Of course, I understand physiology." The twinkle in his eye should have scared me.

My inappropriate use of the term "synovial fluid" led to a battery of tests that defies the imagination for sheer grossness—I think I passed out twice as he was pumping 50 ccs of saline into my joint with a wide-bore needle to see if it leaked out and the membrane surrounding the joint had indeed been punctured. It hadn't.

Take Charge

Medical terms have specific meanings. If you use one, you need to know exactly how the doctor will understand it. Improper use of a term could lead to unnecessary tests or delays in symptom management.

Even if you are not as show-offy as I might be with new words, I bet many of you have done another thing that I am guilty of, which can have equally bad consequences. Raise your hand if you have ever sat and nodded while your doctor was using a term that you didn't understand. You might have thought "I'll look it up later" or "I can figure this out from context," but then you left and completely forgot what the term was. I am always dismayed, but sympathetic, when my family members or friends call and say, "The doctor said that I had this thing that starts with a 'b'—no, wait, it was a 'p'—hold on, I take it back, it definitely started with a 'b' and he said that it might be serious."

It is important—no, *crucial*—to master the vocabulary, terms, and concepts around MS. If you listen to a lawyer or a chef talk, there is a special language that efficiently and accurately communicates concepts in their specific fields. MS has a language, too—a set of terms and concepts that you need to understand in order to think and communicate well about your illness. If you possess the vocabulary, the world of research also opens up to you, as you begin to navigate ideas around immunology and neurology and decode results of treatment trials.

Here are some steps to mastering MS vocabulary and creating an MS encyclopedia. Each day, you will define or explain about five terms or concepts. You can use the Internet or you can refer to books. Once you write out the terms *in your own words* you'll be much closer to understanding and mastering the major concepts around MS.

Take Charge

If you can't use a term naturally, in your own words, and explain it to a friend, then you don't yet have mastery of it. Mastery of a term means you are in control of discussions and communications around that topic. It is beneficial to have mastery of at least some of the most relevant terms to your situation.

Make a list of terms to define. You can keep a running list of terms that you "collect" in your reading about MS. Some terms to get you started are: ataxia, axon, blood-brain barrier, brain atrophy, central nervous system, corticosteroid, demyelination, evoked potentials, expanded disability status scale (EDSS), gadolinium, l'Hermitte's sign, myelin, oligoclonal bands, paresis, paresthesia, plaque, and remission. Make sure to include terms specific to your symptoms or situation that you may need when talking to your doctor, researching clinical trials, or investigating possible treatments.

Schedule time. You'll need to set aside between 15 and 30 minutes every day for about a week for this exercise. Be sure to schedule this time, otherwise it probably won't happen. You could do it while your family is watching TV in the evening. You could do it over your lunch break at work. It doesn't matter when, but you'll need time to work on the definitions.

Gather resources. You may have a book or two on MS—those often have glossaries in the back that can be really helpful. You may also know a few Web sites that are good. (See next section, "Define your questions and get your answers on the Web.")

Use your own words. It will be tempting to just look up the words, read the definitions, and move on—DON'T DO IT. The goal of this whole exercise is for you to have a mastery of these terms. To get that mastery, you need to write them out in your own words. Composing and writing will use more of your brain, which will help you remember the concepts and give you a feeling of expertise and mastery.

You can add to definitions, make them personal, and include observations. If you are writing about a symptom you have, you can focus on your level of severity. Make your MS encyclopedia about you and focus on the things that are most important to you. Don't worry about format. You don't need to write formal definitions—your entries can be notes, lists, or little sketches. Do whatever will help you remember all the details the best. No one needs to see your MS encyclopedia but you, so don't worry about editing and making your entries perfect. Just be sure that you can understand the terms and concepts that you need to know.

Know Your Stuff

Give yourself a little quiz to see if you can answer some questions accurately—for example: Why do your medications work? Why do your symptoms change? Why does MS impact your brain's processing speed?

Try to answer the question "why?" when possible. For example, if you are describing a symptom, try to explain why that symptom occurs. Explain why medications work.

Take your MS encyclopedia further by adding more concepts. Include entries on a variety of related subjects, such as: which kinds of exercise are best for someone with your symptoms, how sleep affects MS, complementary and alternative approaches that may help your symptoms (as well as which ones to avoid), or different tips for dealing with symptoms you may have. Keep making entries in your MS encyclopedia as you run across new terms, new treatments, and new symptoms.

Define Your Questions and Get Your Answers on the Web

For many people, the Internet has become a surrogate friend to whom intimate secrets are told via blogs, a financial advisor to guide us through rocky investment waters, a place where we can meet all sorts of interesting people (including potential future spouses), and a shopping mall with an infinite variety of goods and services, minus parking lots and crowds.

The Internet has also opened up an entire universe of information that, until recently, was only available in medical libraries or stashed away in the brains of researchers and physicians. For those of us with multiple sclerosis, the Internet can be like a "candy store" of information and options that we used to rely on our doctor to transmit to us in annual 20-minute visits. On the other hand, much to the dismay of many medical professionals, the Internet has also become a virtual doctor to many that seek answers and help, as well as prescriptions for those who find their way into the "underground."

Do Your Best

Don't surf the Web for medical information without setting up rules for yourself about how to evaluate the things you find. Otherwise your search for information may end up being frustrating and misleading.

The Internet is wonderful for so many reasons. I write for the Internet (ms.about.com) and I would like to think that my articles have helped my readers navigate confusing situations, calmed them down when something unfamiliar happened, and provided enough background and support to discuss something new with their doctors in a way that gives them answers. Conversely, the Internet can also be not-so-wonderful, and even dangerous. Given the "benefit" of anonymity, anyone can post anything, and, to the casual surfer, completely fabricated diatribes can look just like recommendations based on data coming out of peer-reviewed trials. Often, the more upset or alternative or convinced that people are about something, the more they write about it and the "bigger" it can get on the Internet. Given these potential information "detours" that people can be led down, it helps to have some guidelines in place when looking for answers on the World Wide Web.

Here are some steps for surfing the medical Web:

We love the NIH. The National Institutes of Health (NIH) is a tremendous institution, and an excellent place to start any health-related search, as many other sites "adapt" their information from the NIH pages. The NIH has compiled information on different diseases and conditions, as well as on all prescription medications, over-the-counter drugs, and herbs and supplements and their uses on a Web site called MedlinePlus (www.medlineplus.gov). It sponsors (via Congress) much of the medical research that takes place in the United States. Go there and read about MS symptoms, treatment, financial matters, diagnosis, research, and many other topics. MedlinePlus also has links to other sites such as the Mayo Clinic, the National Multiple Sclerosis Society, and the various institutes within the NIH. Although all of the sources found here are reliable, not all of the information is always in total agreement or emphasizes the same things, so definitely read from more than one source when looking for answers.

The Real World

Most people, even many physicians, don't know much about MS. You need broad knowledge to assess what you read yourself.

Conduct a basic search. When searching for information, there is a fine line between being too specific and not being specific enough. You need to come up with a keyword that an author would have featured prominently in his or her writing. You also need to think about whether your search needs to be specific to MS or not. For example, you might find some great suggestions about fatigue from sites about other illnesses. You'll need to keep experimenting and trying to put yourself in the mind of the writer. When searching about MS, write out the words "multiple sclerosis." If you just search "MS," you'll end up with lots of unhelpful results about Microsoft products, *Ms. Magazine*, and the state of Mississippi. Generally, you should search using the keywords "multiple sclerosis," combined with an additional term that you want information about, such as "numbness."

Read the address. In your search results, at the bottom of each entry that appears, is the actual address of the site. It will look like this: www.nmss.org. Before clicking on a link, read the address of the site. Look for familiar words from respected places such as Harvard, the Mayo Clinic, the Cleveland Clinic, or the National Multiple Sclerosis

Society in the address. If an address ends in ".gov," then you can be sure it is a government Web site. If the address ends in ".edu," then you know it is an academic or university Web site. Addresses that end in ".org" are likely, but not always, nonprofit Web sites.

Learn how to use bookmarks. If you don't use bookmarks, you might be missing an important feature of your Internet browser. Bookmarks allow you to make a list of pages that you like. You can create folders and put the bookmarks in them. As you find interesting or helpful sites, you just click and add the bookmarks. For instance, you could create a folder labeled "fatigue ideas," which may contain links to articles about tips to conserve energy, discussions of different medications prescribed to help people with MS-related fatigue, and an online discussion group of people with MS writing about fatigue. Using bookmarks really speeds up surfing and helps you retrace your steps. If you don't already use bookmarks, read about them in the help section of your browser or ask someone to explain them to you.

Check your dates. Pay attention to when an article was written and the last time it was updated. This information is usually at the bottom of the page, but could appear anywhere. Keep in mind that for MS, many things changed when the disease-modifying medications were approved in the mid-1990s. It is likely that anything written before that will be very out-of-date. Sometimes, dates will not be on Web sites— just do your best to assess when things when things were written.

Medical review matters. Some Web sites will mention that the content was reviewed by a doctor or medically reviewed. This means that a doctor read through the information on the site and certified that it is correct from a medical standpoint. Look for that, especially when a site is giving medical or treatment advice.

Do Your Best

Be fair when you search. Don't simply search until you find the information that you think you want. Many people use the Internet as a crutch to justify their decisions. Instead, make your searches about finding facts, not opinions that you like or agree with.

Conduct a site search. One of the handiest ways to find information is to conduct a site search. In Google, you simply type *site:sitename.com search term* (replacing *sitename.com* with the address of the site you want to search, and replacing *search term* with the keywords that you are interested in). Google will return search results only for that site. For example, if you are interested in information about fatigue from the National Multiple Sclerosis Society, but don't want to spend a lot of time clicking through links, you could try the following search in Google: *site:www.nmss.org fatigue.* If you were interested in learning more about a particular medication, such as Copaxone, from MedlinePlus, you could type the following search into Google: *site:www.medlineplus.gov copaxone.* Remember to place a colon after the word "site," and a space after the Web site address.

Narrow it down. Sometimes you have a question about tips to deal with side effects of a medication, a problem related to a symptom that you are experiencing, or something else specific. Go ahead and type in the specific question. Then click on all the links that are returned. Don't worry about where the information is coming from at this point. You'll probably find a forum or a blog where someone with MS is writing about the same problem you have. This is good. There are often very helpful suggestions and practical information on these types of sites. You may even find some people to write to and ask directly. Just remember, this may not be medical information, but information from people like you who are trying to deal with their MS on a daily basis. That doesn't mean it isn't helpful, just don t do anything drastic without talking to your doctor.

Tips for surfing the medical Web:

- Find 5 to 10 really reliable Web sites that you can trust. Start your searches for information there. Make MedlinePlus one of them.

- Find 3 to 5 sites written by people with MS. They may be blog-type sites or discussion-based sites. Hang out there for a few days and see if there is interesting support or information available. Just don't get caught up in people's ranting. When someone is upset about something these days, they write about it and post it on the Internet.

- Don't shop when searching for medical information. You will run across all sorts of ads and products that people are trying to sell you. Assume they are all scams. Don't buy anything.

- Stay focused—write down the information you are looking for and try to stick to it, otherwise you could get lost and end up spending too much time at the computer.

- Stay on the reliable and trustworthy Web sites, at least until you have a mastery of the topics and concepts.

- Read any "worst-case scenario" or "miracle cure" stories with caution. There are extreme cases of every disease, and MS is no exception. These stories are often found on the Internet, as are claims that MS is caused or made worse by all sorts of things that we come into contact with every day. Don't let these stories or theories add to your stress or lead you to make extreme changes in your lifestyle without talking to your doctor. Do not, under any circumstances, ever change anything about your medication, including stopping it or changing dosages, based on something you read on the Internet (or anywhere else).

The Bottom Line

Based on personal observations, I would guess that about 85% of people, upon receiving a new electronic gadget, tear open the box and start pushing buttons before reading even the first page of the instruction manual. I have appliances that I have had for years that have blinking lights that I don't understand or a time panel that has been flashing "00:00" since I plugged it in.

Take Charge

As a person living with MS, you simply must put in lots of research and learning time. Knowledge is what will give you as much control over your situation as possible. Knowledge will also make the unknown future much less scary.

We cannot afford to be this way with our bodies, especially those of us living with MS. We have to be able to identify what is going on with us in order to know when to take action and what kind of action to take. Then we need to be able to talk to our doctors about it, so that they have the information that they need to help us. Only by having some ideas about what it means when certain things are happening to us can we fight the fear of the unknown and create a plan based on knowledge rather than emotion.

3

Put Your Symptoms in Their Place

For all of our talk about the various challenges of living with multiple sclerosis, let's face it—most of our troubles originate with our symptoms and how they impact our lives. I might be bothered on some intellectual level if I knew that I was losing brain volume at a fairly rapid rate, but if I didn't have a whole mess of symptoms to confirm it and an underlying dread of increased future disability, I probably wouldn't be as motivated to give myself a daily injection.

Take Charge

I hope you don't have many of the symptoms described in this chapter, but it is helpful to know about possible symptoms that might pop up in your future and identify weird sensations that might be bugging you right now. Read this chapter carefully and refer to it if you feel something new. By being able to identify something as possibly linked to your MS, you will be able to calmly come up with a strategy rather than panic.

Multiple sclerosis is often referred to as the disease with the most symptoms. The vast number of possible symptoms is complicated by the fact that not only can any of them appear at any time, one never knows how severe they will get or how long they will last. When I get a new symptom or one of my existing symptoms acts up, I have to fight the tendency to automatically assume that this is it—I will feel like this forever, or that I will continue to feel worse on a steep and swift decline. For this reason, among others, it helps to learn as much about the symptom as possible and to figure out what my options are before indulging in panic or fatalism about the future.

As people living with MS, it is crucial that we understand, but don't overreact to, the symptoms that we might encounter. Clearly, it is instinctive to focus on the current physical manifestations of MS and fret about how bad a symptom might get or what might be coming next. But our energy is used much better to figure out how to decrease the discomfort and interference with our activities as much as we can, and to incorporate whatever we can't fix (symptom-wise) into our lives, rather than living in servitude to these symptoms.

This chapter will provide basic information about many of the symptoms associated with MS. The goal is to help you identify any symptom that you might be having, give you a heads-up as to how the symptom might affect your life, and provide basic information about strategies to "fight back" against these symptoms—for instance, whether prescription medications might help, if physical therapy might have some benefits, and any simple measures that you might be able to try at home for relief. This overview is intended as a catalyst to get you started on more in-depth research about what you are experiencing and on your quest to feel better. Also, please be aware that you may have symptoms that do not appear on this list that are still part of MS and, on a more positive note, there will surely be many symptoms in this chapter that you will never experience.

Fatigue

Fatigue is one of the biggest things that separate those of us with MS from those people with intact myelin. An estimated 85 to 95% of people with MS experience the unbelievable, crushing fatigue that is impossible to explain to anyone who hasn't been there. It is described by many MSers, including people in wheelchairs, as their most debilitating symptom. Sounds about right to me.

Fatigue in MS is caused by many factors, which can be grouped into those causing primary fatigue and secondary fatigue. Primary fatigue is the result of the disease process itself, and is caused by demyelination in the central nervous system. In most cases, we are talking about "lassitude," an overwhelming tiredness that is not directly related to increased activity. It can be increased by hot or humid weather or by raising the body temperature through exercise or exertion, but mostly it is just *there*, hanging out—insidious and defying all attempts to banish it. Not to be overlooked is a form of primary fatigue called "short-circuiting" or "localized" fatigue, in which affected nerves of individual muscle groups tire with use, such as your legs after walking or your hand after writing.

Secondary fatigue is not caused directly by the MS disease process itself, but is a result of living with all these other symptoms and trying constantly to compensate for abilities we used to have and just live normal lives. For instance, many of us experience sleep disturbances that clearly can exacerbate fatigue. These lost hours of sleep may be the result of MS symptoms such as spasms, depression or anxiety, pain, the frequent need to urinate at night (nocturia), or medications that interfere with sleep, like Solu-Medrol. Then there are many medications that directly cause fatigue, including those taken specifically for MS, such as the disease-modifying therapies that are made from beta-interferon (Avonex, Betaseron, and Rebif), Tysabri, and Novantrone, as well as some medications taken for MS symptoms such as spasticity or pain. Let's not forget the fatigue-inducing drugs that we take for conditions unrelated to our MS, including medications for high-blood pressure, allergy medications and others containing antihistamines, and anti-anxiety drugs.

As those of us with MS go through our days doing everyday things, we are constantly trying to compensate for our damaged nerves. I've heard that for someone with MS to do something, even something very simple—such as moving one hand a couple of inches—requires up to 5 times more brain activity than the same action done by someone without MS. That's because we need to make up for missing neural connections that have been lost as a result of demyelination and atrophy. Thinking of all the things we do all day, it is no wonder that we are fatigued from the exertion needed to move all our parts, much less the constant need to compensate for symptoms like spasticity or muscle weakness, which may make it harder to walk, maintain our balance, or complete tasks around the house.

Take Charge
We can't control our fatigue, but we can control how we react to it.

There is also an interesting (in a horrific kind of way) relationship between depression and fatigue. Depression often causes people to feel overwhelmingly tired. In some people, the fatigue itself causes depression. Some of the medications used to treat depression can also cause fatigue.

Then, of course, we come to the things that affect everyone, simply because they are human, but that are worse in those of us with MS. Lack of proper nutrition can cause swings in blood sugar, leading to general tiredness. Infections, such as colds, flu, or urinary tract infections may cause fatigue in people without MS, but can make us feel like we have been hit by a train. Then there is the insidiously frustrating cycle of lack of physical fitness contributing to fatigue, but the fatigue often making exercise seem a near-impossibility.

What Fatigue Feels Like and How It Can Affect Your Life

Describing MS-related fatigue to someone who hasn't been there is like trying to describe the color blue to a person who was born blind. The closest description that I have been able to muster was to compare it to having a nasty hangover and jetlag at the same time. To break it down more precisely, MS-related fatigue often has specific characteristics which make it different than other types of "tiredness" or "exhaustion." It occurs daily and may be present in the morning, even after a good night's sleep, but tends to get worse later in the day. It can also come on suddenly, especially in the presence of heat and humidity. For some people (like me), there are additional related symptoms, including a feeling of heaviness in the arms and legs; worsening of other symptoms, such as problems with balance or vision, or slurred speech; difficulty concentrating; vertigo, dizziness, or nausea; headaches; and flu-like symptoms. You can be "officially" diagnosed as having MS-related fatigue if you have fatigue symptoms for at least 50% of the time, lasting for more than 6 weeks.

I'll say it. Fatigue sucks. For me, it is the worst thing about having MS, as it makes *everything* so much harder. Symptoms that I could deal with in isolation (as if that ever happens) have a symbiotic relationship with my fatigue—they all love each other and feed off of each other in a terrible dance. For example, my cognitive dysfunction is worse on the days that I wake up fatigued, which is about 50% of the time during the warmer months. This causes me stress, which makes the fatigue feel worse, which makes me panic—the cycle continues like this until I can "reset" with a nap or a 5-minute shutdown with my head on the table, which delivers me back to a barely functional state.

Do not underestimate fatigue. Fatigue can steal your physical energy and leave you unable to perform basic daily tasks, much less hold down a full-time job. It can also affect you emotionally and drain you of optimism and enthusiasm.

Fight Back Against Fatigue

I really would love to tell you that fatigue can be fixed. I really would. I can't. But I can tell you that, although fatigue might hang on, your attitude toward it can make a huge difference in your quality of life. Imagine that you are standing in the ocean in water up to your chest. The waves are coming and you can face them down defiantly and angrily, palms outstretched, only to get knocked on your butt. Or you can soften your knees and float with the waves, up and down, until you find your footing again. In the case of fatigue, "fighting back" may mean learning how to work around your enemy, rather than going on the offensive.

Entire books have been written about the subject of managing MS-related fatigue. In strategizing ways to lessen your fatigue, it is important to identify contributing factors, such as medications, sleep problems, poor diet, use of alcohol, and other things that you can directly influence. It is also key that you can describe your fatigue accurately to your doctor, because it will help her figure out which actions to take and how aggressive to be in treating fatigue. (See "How to talk to your doctor about your symptoms" in this chapter.) The first thing that might be tried is to adjust the dosages or timing of medications (or switch drugs altogether) that may contribute to fatigue by directly making you tired or by interfering with sleep. Another approach is to prescribe medications to help you sleep, if insomnia is a problem. Your doctor might also ask you some questions to determine if you are depressed.

The Real World

Fatigue is lonely—no one can see it. Work hard to make sure those around you understand, as much as possible, what MS fatigue is and the effect it has on your life.

Because exertion is a factor in fatigue, your doc might prescribe physical therapy to help you strengthen your muscles and build stamina or occupational therapy to help you learn to streamline your actions so that they use less energy. He might also suggest that you make adjustments to your home to make things easier. Your doctor will also be interested in any sort of infection you may have, so make sure you mention any urinary tract discomfort or respiratory symptoms.

In terms of drugs to treat fatigue, your options are pretty limited. Some people find that drugs like Provigil and Amantidine work wonders, others (like me) find that the side effects overshadow any benefits. If your doctor is willing to experiment, he might try Fampridine (4-AP), low dose naltrexone, or Adderall (a drug used to treat attention-deficit hyperactivity disorder)—all of which have been used with success in some people with MS.

Depression

There is a very complicated relationship between depression and MS. MS can cause depression as a result of the disease process itself, and people can also get depressed from the emotional burden of dealing with MS or its symptoms, reactions of friends and loved ones, and fear of the unknown. It can also be caused or made worse as a side effect to certain drugs used to treat MS (such as Betaseron and Avonex), and a course of Solu-Medrol can cause periods of hyperactivity and euphoria, followed by a "letdown" period. Depression also has many of the same symptoms as MS (fatigue, cognitive disturbances, headaches), which makes it difficult to determine which problem to target first. At least half of the people living with MS have symptoms of depression at some point in their lives, and it is estimated that at any given time 14% of people with MS are depressed.

What Depression Feels Like and How It Can Affect Your Life

According to the *Diagnostic and Statistical Manual of Mental Disorders, fourth edition (DSM-IV)*, the diagnostic manual of the American Psychiatric Association that contains the criteria used by mental health professionals to diagnose people, you are clinically depressed if you have had at least five of the following symptoms, representing a change in function, for at least two weeks: sadness, loss of interest in things you previously liked to do, change in appetite, problems sleeping, moving faster or slower than usual (so that people notice), fatigue, feelings of guilt, cognitive problems, or suicidal thoughts. In addition, the symptoms must be severe enough to upset your daily routine, seriously impair your work, or interfere with your relationships and cannot be part of a normal reaction to the death of a loved one.[1]

The Real World

While depressed, you may not have the insight to realize that you are depressed. Be sure a loved one whom you talk with frequently knows the signs of depression and what to do about it.

According to the *DSM-IV*, clinical depression does not have a specific cause like alcohol, drugs, medication side effects, or physical illness. But for those of us with MS and for those who treat us, this is confusing, because MS *does* cause depression as part of the disease process, and it can be a side effect of some of the MS disease-modifying therapies or other medications. Further complicating matters, you may also feel or experience uncontrollable crying, irritability, unexplained aches and pains, stomachaches and digestive problems, decreased sex drive, or headaches—many of which are also symptoms of MS.

Like other symptoms, there is a spectrum of depression—people who are on one end may just feel sluggish and less enthusiastic about some things. On the other end of the spectrum, depression can be debilitating, and untreated depression can lead to suicide. Studies show that people with MS are between 2 and 7.5 times as likely to commit suicide as people in the general population.

Fight Back Against Depression

Depression is particularly evil, as it can mercilessly target and erode the very resolve that you need in order to fight it. The pain can be worse than physical pain and just as immobilizing. Remember, depression is not your fault. It is not a sign of weakness, and nothing to be embarrassed about, however, you must fight it if it comes. You have no choice.

Whether you meet all of the necessary criteria for depression or not, or if you think some of them are just part of having MS, it doesn't matter in terms of what you need to do next. If you have MS and feel very sad or have no interest in things around you, you absolutely need to seek help as soon as possible. Leave the diagnosis and treatment to a professional. By "professional," I do not mean a chiropractor, nutritionist, apitherapist, aromatherapist, or reflexologist. Although any physician can prescribe antidepressant medications, I HIGHLY recommend that you see a psychiatrist for any suspected depression. Start with your doctor or call your local MS Society Chapter for recommendations for a psychiatrist.

The treatment of depression requires careful monitoring and individualized treatment plans. A psychiatrist has experience with all forms of depression and has observed the effects of different medications firsthand. She will be able to tell you what to expect and ask the right questions to allow her to adjust your dose over time to ensure the best response possible. Even more specifically, it is important to see a psychiatrist used to treating people with MS, because depression symptoms must be "untangled" from similar MS symptoms, in order to determine the best course of treatment. Your disease-modifying therapy or symptom management medications may need to be changed if they are contributing to the problem. There are many medications that are effective against depression, but often it is a matter of trial and error before exactly the right combination and dosages are determined. Research has shown that combining medications with psychotherapy (talk therapy) is the most effective treatment of depression. Depending on what is available in your area and what you are comfortable with, this can be in the form of individual, one-on-one sessions or in a group setting.

I'll say it again—it is important that you get help to feel better. All of us living with MS have more than enough to deal with, and depression can affect our physical health because it can influence how well or poorly we take care of ourselves.

Cognitive Dysfunction

Cognitive dysfunction may be the MS symptom that makes me the saddest. I can get angry at my constantly tingling feet and frustrated with my lack of coordination or trembling hands, but being mad at how my

esting—it is 90 degrees out here," and go about my business, only
alize several minutes later that all my systems are slowing down
feel like I am hearing and seeing things through a blanket as my
ments feel like I am swimming in wet concrete.

at intolerance is such a common symptom that people used to
gnosed with MS based on the results of a "hot bath test." Because
ows down nerve impulse transmission along already-damaged
increased symptoms will show up when the body's core tem-
e increases by as little as one-quarter to a half degree.

t Intolerance Feels Like and How It Can Affect Your Life

lerance in MS shows up as a "pseudoexacerbation," the expe-
having symptoms appear or worsen due to heat exposure.
any MS symptom can be much worse in the heat, the most
ones to act up are: decreased cognitive function, numbness
g in the feet, fatigue, blurred vision, tremor, and weakness.
, symptoms appear that we might not have felt before,
result of a past lesion that was slight enough or positioned
at it did not cause a relapse or symptoms dramatic enough
or instance, Uhthoff's sign refers to blurred vision as a
at exposure and is caused by a lesion on the optic nerve,
ople experiencing Uhthoff's sign never had classic symp-
neuritis.
exacerbation is different than a true relapse. In the case
acerbation, when the body's temperature returns to nor-
mptoms begin to disappear. No damage, such as inflam-
elination or new lesions, has occurred during these
ations.
nly tell you that many, many of us with MS have to limit
hot weather. This is often not as simple as choosing to
ly vacation in the mountains rather than on the beach.
lace that gets hot at least part of the year, summers
ou are under "lockdown," not able to go places with
outside with your children, or enjoy normal warm
s. For some MSers, heat intolerance can be debilitat
hey are unable to function well at even slightly ele
es and must consider moving to a cooler geographi

own brain has slowed down and how my thought patterns are misfiring
is a little too complicated. Cognitive dysfunction is also the symptom
that is the hardest for me to talk about with people without MS,
because it often comes across as a lame-sounding apology for being
"ditzy" or is met with people mentioning how forgetful they, too, have
become since they had children or turned 75. Between 34 and 65% of
people with MS have some sort of cognitive impairment, although for
some people the symptoms might be so subtle that they went unno-
ticed or were attributed to other things, such as aging or being tired.

What Cognitive Dysfunction Feels Like and How It Can Affect Your Life

Like every other MS symptom, cognitive dysfunction manifests differently in everyone and can change daily or even hourly. Short-term
memory is often affected, resulting in situations like forgetting whose
telephone number you just dialed or standing in front of an open refrigerator without a clue what you originally were going to get. One of my
darkest moments was forgetting which of my infant twins had received
her dose of powerful antibiotics as I held the second dose in my hand,
bewildered.

> ### Know Your Stuff
>
> Cognitive symptoms are often overlooked by the people experi-
> encing them. A good understanding of the cognitive symptoms of
> MS may help you make sense of many difficulties that cause you
> to be frustrated with yourself.

Cognitive dysfunction can impede us in many other ways, as well.
Carrying on a conversation may be very difficult as you find yourself
repeating a sentence or part of a story to someone to whom you just
told it. You may also have word-finding difficulties that hamper being
able to communicate precisely. Following (much less participating in)
a complex discussion may also be challenging, especially if several
people are talking or if the topic changes often. Your judgment when
trying to solve problems may be impaired, as you might find that you
get easily overwhelmed if something is too complex, because it is hard
to organize thoughts and tasks, to apply lessons learned from multiple
past experiences, and to be "flexible" enough in your thinking to come

up with alternate solutions if things don't go as you had planned. You might also find that you are unable to multitask or that even minor ambient noise, like the television or music, can make it virtually impossible to concentrate on things like reading or performing sequential tasks, like those involved in cooking.

Your brain may simply not be able to take in quickly and prioritize all of the information coming in at once, resulting in slower speed of information processing. This may manifest as problems processing spoken or written language, sensory information, spatial information (like that involved in navigating while driving), or more abstract things, like social cues and reading people's emotions.

Do Your Best

Many components of cognitive dysfunction can be managed. Make lists, write things down obsessively, and avoid situations requiring snap decisions.

The good news about MS-related cognitive dysfunction is that it very rarely progresses to real, debilitating dementia. This only occurs in less than 5% of people with multiple sclerosis; these individuals are usually very severely affected by other symptoms as well. The bad news is that cognitive problems in people with MS can become severe enough to make it difficult to work in a profession that requires speedy or complex problem-solving. Jeffrey Gingold describes working as an attorney in his book, *Facing The Cognitive Challenges of Multiple Sclerosis*:

> "My thoughts began to drag, and it was difficult to absorb even the simplest information. My mind was busy with: *focus on sitting up straight, keep eyes wide-open, lift both knees to avoid drop-foot stumbling, and show a confident smile.* It was a strained balance, perhaps similar to trying to hand-write federal legislation while scuba-diving on a half-tank of air and watching for sharks."[2]

I know that cognitive dysfunction has robbed me of some of my confidence. I used to be comfortable in almost any social situation, but I now find myself second-guessing things that I say or staying quiet to avoid repeating myself or using the wrong word. I have also virtually

stopped driving, due to anxiety about forgetting the rou paying attention to what I was doing, and overall dread a terrible accident—all as a result of my brain not be with all the microdecisions required to safely mane

Fight Back Against Cognitive Dysfunction

Cognitive dysfunction and fatigue certainly fe one overall strategy might be to plan activiti sharpness to take place during your "good" ti environment and relationships to be as calr clutter, turn off sources of noise, and make your house. When having a conversation ir don't hesitate to ask people to repeat them ing the conversation and to confirm impe anything else that needs to be exact. Don't you need time to think something over important, rather than making a hasty de to someone or doing anything else, foc what you are trying to do, rather than make a grocery list, and file your finger

Get yourself organized in a way t you can find things without using up for something, then getting flustered ting what you were looking for in t versation with your brain, thinking tempted to run off and play with e focusing on the task at hand. Rem accomplish, and be imaginative three ingredients that you nee keys" over and over with a fu Promise yourself treats (Skitt) plish your task. Whatever it ta

H

There are times that I go o sun hits me and the tingle there are situations wher

Do Your Best

Make a strategy for staying cool. Get a disabled parking placard to park close to stores and work, don't get in a blazing hot car (have someone turn the car on first and run the air conditioner before you get in) and think through other ways to avoid letting your body heat up.

I can tell you that when it is hot outside, no matter how cool I am able to get inside, I still have to be careful cooking over a hot stove or taking clothes out of a hot dryer. I get dizzy and confused and have experienced scary symptoms.

Deaths have even been reported among people with MS who were sunbathing or relaxing in hot tubs and presumably lost the ability to get out of the heat.

Fight Back Against Heat Intolerance

The bottom line is to keep cool, starting with your environment. If you live in a hot climate, air conditioning will be essential, the cost of which might be tax-deductible with a doctor's prescription. We tinted all the windows in our house, which went a long way toward cutting our electricity bill (30% in summer months) and gives the house a calm, cool feeling inside. You can also cool down your environment and expand your territory with outdoor misting fans, which blow a fine mist of water into the air and can lower temperatures in the immediate area by 20 degrees.

Don't Panic

Often, people with MS confuse heat intolerance with a relapse. Get cool and see what happens before "going there" in your mind.

The other approach to take after bringing down the heat in your environment is to bring down the heat in your body. Start with preventing situations that expose you to excessive heat. This does not (necessarily) mean staying inside with the shades drawn. Instead, begin by getting "the tag," aka a disabled parking placard, so that you can avoid crossing those endless, shimmering-with-heat parking lots in the summer.

Next, focus on actually bringing your core temperature down by applying cold. Starting with the simplest (and cheapest) ideas, you can reduce your core temperature by drinking ice-cold beverages—try keeping a couple of plastic bottles filled with water or iced tea in your freezer to drink as they melt. If you know you are going outside, pre-cool yourself by taking a cold shower, which can buy you some time in the heat. Don't wear socks! If you are lucky enough to have access to a pool, consider taking up residence in it during the hot times. More expensive options involve looking into the large variety of personal cooling products available, including different types of vests, neck-bands, and hats. The Multiple Sclerosis Association of America has a Cooling Distribution Program to get these products to people with MS who cannot afford them.

Bladder Dysfunction

In the interest of continuing to bring you news about MS symptoms that you either have or can look forward to, I'll tell you that bladder dysfunction occurs in at least 80% of us, with estimates that up to 96% of people who have had MS for more than 10 years will experience uri-nary problems at some point. Oh, goody.

Bladder dysfunction in MS happens when nerve signals to the blad-der and urinary sphincter (the muscles surrounding the opening to the bladder) are blocked or delayed because of lesions on the spinal cord. The dysfunction can occur for two reasons: the bladder is spastic, so it isn't holding the urine, or the bladder isn't emptying all the way, because the sphincter is spastic (contracting when it is supposed to be relaxing to let out the urine, or vice versa).

What Bladder Dysfunction Feels Like and How It Can Affect Your Life

Bladder dysfunction can take several forms. Hesitancy describes an urge to urinate, but it takes a long time to begin to urinate or it is diffi-cult to keep the urine flowing. Sometimes, the attempt is even "dry," meaning no urine is released at all. Urgency is a different problem, where the need to urinate comes on suddenly and strongly and may be accompanied by an uncomfortable "full" feeling in the bladder. Frequency means there is a need to urinate much more often than usual, although often there is very little or no urine released. This often happens at night (called "nocturia"), causing sleep disturbances. Incontinence can either feel like a sudden urge to urinate, followed by the flow starting immediately before there is a chance to react, or dribbling or leaking with no warning or sensation.

Do Your Best

The bladder-sleep connection cannot be underestimated. A bout of bladder dysfunction can have you waking up dozens of times during the night (my all-time record was 39 times in one night), resulting in terrible sleep and adding to your fatigue the next day. Try different strategies to keep your bladder behaving, rather than just trying to live with this symptom.

Regardless of which way your bladder decides to misbehave, the biggest impact of bladder dysfunction is often psychological distress. Many people find the whole situation embarrassing to the point of completely avoiding social situations. People often stop leaving their house and stop having sex.

Untreated bladder dysfunction can cause permanent damage to the urinary tract when there is incomplete emptying of the bladder and urine is retained. This can result in both urinary tract infections and formation of bladder stones from accumulated minerals. Constantly leaking urine can result in skin breakdown and infection.

Fight Back Against Bladder Dysfunction

The good news is that most bladder dysfunction is treatable, or at least can be managed so that you can do things that you enjoy without constantly worrying about leaking or having to run to find a bathroom. The initial step in treatment is to have the condition evaluated by a physician. The first test will probably be to determine if a urinary tract infection is the culprit—these are very common among people with MS due to urine retention and can cause many of the symptoms mentioned, as well as possibly lead to an MS relapse if untreated. If a test is positive, the infection will be treated with antibiotics and you will watch to see if the symptoms disappear. If you do not have a UTI, it is likely that you will take a variety of tests that make up a "urodynamic assessment," which may be necessary to determine appropriate treatments.

Depending on what type of bladder dysfunction you may have, there are several medications that might help. Antispasticity agents may be used to relax the sphincter muscle. There are also drugs to promote the flow of urine, drugs to reduce bladder spasms and drugs to reduce the amount of urine made by the kidneys. You may be taught to perform intermittent self-catheterization, which is the insertion of a thin tube into the bladder to allow the urine to flow out. Not only does this really work, many people find that their bladder function becomes more normal after doing this for weeks or months. If medications don't help you or if you have difficulties with self-catheterization, there are surgeries that can help, including having an electrical device (similar to a pacemaker) implanted to stimulate the sacral nerves.

There are a number of things that you do to ensure that your medications or other approaches have the best chance of working against bladder dysfunction. One approach involves regulating and timing fluid intake, as well as urinating on a regular schedule, rather than waiting for the urge. Certain beverages may also make your problems worse, so you may want to experiment with restricting your intake of caffeine, alcohol, and orange juice. It is important that you *not* restrict overall intake of fluid, as this can lead to urinary tract infections or constipation. Some people find that drinking unsweetened cranberry juice daily will help prevent urinary tract infections.

Spasticity

Though most experts estimate that about 20% of people with MS experience some degree of spasticity at some point, there is evidence that up to one-third of people with multiple sclerosis alter their daily activities because of spasticity. Spasticity is best understood as an increase in muscle tone, which means the muscles do not relax as much or as easily as they should, affecting movement.

What Spasticity Feels Like and How It Can Affect Your Life

It probably comes as no surprise that spasticity is primarily caused by demyelination. Due to the resulting slow or interrupted nerve impulses, the muscles may malfunction in three ways: not relax as quickly as they should, tighten involuntarily, or stay contracted for long periods of time (or constantly, in some cases). These "glitches" lead to different types of spasticity. Extensor spasms cause the limb to jerk away from the body—this usually affects the quadriceps (the large muscles on the front of the thigh), causing the lower leg to straighten.

Flexor spasms almost always affect the legs, especially the hamstrings or hip flexors, and cause the leg to contract, or bend, toward the body. Clonus is when muscles jerk or twitch repeatedly, most commonly seen when the foot taps rapidly and repetitively on the floor or the knee or ankle jerk repeatedly after stimulation (such as tapping at the joint), rather than the normal response of one tap or jerk. Adductor spasms cause a person's legs to close together tightly, making it difficult to separate them.

Several things can aggravate spasticity, acting as a trigger for spasms—these things are called "noxious stimuli" and can include infections, such as respiratory, urinary tract, or bladder infections; pain; sores or skin breakdown; an increase in internal temperature due to fever or exertion; a full bladder; binding or otherwise irritating clothes; constipation; poor posture; stress, worry or anxiety; or extreme environmental temperatures.

For many people, spasticity can be an annoyance or a passing problem that hinders smooth walking one day, but is absent the next. Mild spasticity may be perceived as stiffness, and can cause problems walking with an even gait or using your fingers to perform delicate movements, such as writing or typing. It may just be that walking quickly or climbing stairs is harder than it was previously. Others may actually benefit from mild spasticity or stiffness, as it can counteract some degree of muscle weakness and make it easier to stand.

For some people, however, severe forms of spasticity can cause a problem with mobility, as walking becomes difficult or impossible. Some extensor spasms can be so sudden and strong that they cause a person to fall out of a chair or bed. Flexor spasms can cause limbs to be held in painful positions leading to secondary joint pain.

Fight Back Against Spasticity

Mild problems with spasticity may be greatly helped by eliminating some of the triggers (noxious stimuli) mentioned above. Also, many people find that their spasticity responds well to different complementary and alternative approaches, including yoga, acupuncture, reflexology, biofeedback, massage, Tai Chi, and others.

However, if spasticity is severe enough to interfere with daily activities, it is time to see the doctor. Non-drug interventions that may be tried alone or in combination with medications include physical therapy in the form of stretching, either passively (a therapist stretches the person's limbs) or actively (the person performs the stretching exercises), or hydrotherapy (exercising in water). Mechanical aids, such as braces, may also be used to keep limbs straight.

Pharmaceutical options are usually very effective against spasticity, although many of the medications used can worsen fatigue. The oral medications, which will probably be tried first, depending on the type and severity of the spasms, include: baclofen, different classes of antispasticity and antiseizure drugs, as well as some antihistamines, medications to treat Parkinson's disease, and benzodiazepines. Many people find relief and regain mobility from intrathecal baclofen, whereby the drug is injected into the space in the spinal column containing cerebrospinal fluid via an implanted pump. Botox is frequently used for treating small muscles or areas. More permanent options, which are typically reserved for more severe cases, involve chemical blocks of phenol injected into the muscles of the legs and surgery to sever affected nerves.

Pain, Including MS Hug and Trigeminal Neuralgia

In case you haven't noticed, multiple sclerosis can be very painful. In fact, for many of us with MS, it is difficult to believe that as recently as the 1980s, MS was considered a painless condition. I have been struggling to figure out how or why anyone could make that claim, as pain—in many different forms—has been one of the worst manifestations of my MS. It is estimated that around 80% of people with MS experience MS-related pain at some point, and the National Multiple Sclerosis Society estimates that up to half of us are plagued by chronic pain.

We all have our good days and our bad days. For me, the good days are the ones where I don't have a symptom that was bad enough to be memorable a week later, as opposed to just those kinds of yucky ones that I have learned to live with. I can say that some of my pain symptoms have seared themselves into my memory so well that I can remember them years later, including the specific circumstances of where I was and what was going on when I felt that degree of pain.

Take Charge

Many docs will not recognize pain as a symptom of MS, but it is. If your doctor refuses to listen and strategize different pain solutions with you, then it might be time for a new doctor.

Since my MS diagnosis, I have experienced excruciating "hard-to-catch-my-breath" pain from the MS hug; deep, dull aches in my legs resulting from attempts to adjust my gait to sensory ataxia; severe dysesthesia, as well as allodynia episodes where my clothes touching my legs felt like stinging insects; and "screaming-out-loud" (literally) pain when moving my eyes during a bout of optic neuritis.

Nobody without MS would think to include sources of what I would call "tertiary" MS pain in a discussion of pain as a symptom of MS—still, because of MS, I have fallen, run into doors, and bumped my hips on tables. I have cut myself badly and spilled hot coffee on myself when my hands were shaking. I suppose it would be a stretch to include the pain from injections and infusions, confinement in MRI tubes, or side effects from Solu-Medrol in this list, but all of these things hurt, too.

What MS-Related Pain Feels Like and How It Can Affect Your Life

Pain in MS is complicated. It can fall into one or more of the following categories: neuropathic pain, musculoskeletal (or secondary) pain, or paroxysmal pain. Neuropathic pain is the most common kind of pain in MS and is caused by the demyelination of the disease process itself. It can be explained as follows: Nociceptors are nerve endings that specifically detect painful stimuli. When demyelination occurs, nerve signals traveling along nerve cells may get misdirected to nearby nociceptors, which mistakenly communicate pain signals to the brain. Neuropathic pain symptoms include: paresthesia (numbness and tingling); allodynia (pain as a result of a stimulus), and dysesthesia (a normal stimulus, such as a light touch, is perceived as being painful); trigeminal neuralgia; the "MS hug;" headaches; and optic neuritis.

Musculoskeletal or secondary pain is usually a result of the symptoms of MS, such as spasticity, weakness, immobility or problems walking, and not the disease process itself. Some examples of this are joint pain of the hips and knees due to imbalance and change in gait; stiffness due to immobility; back pain, which can be the result of an unsteady gait, immobility, trying to adapt to the annoying feeling of the MS hug, sitting for extended periods in wheelchairs, or any constant adjustment in movement or position as a result of MS symptoms; pain from flexor spasms, which cause a limb to contract, or bend, toward the body.

Paroxysmal pain refers to pain that has an acute (or sudden) onset, stays for just a couple of seconds or minutes, then fades rapidly or disappears completely (although there may be residual or lingering pain after the episode). Painful paroxysmal symptoms include: trigeminal neuralgia, extensor spasms, and L'Hermitte's sign, the electric-shock type of sensation that runs down the spine when the head is bent forward.

Two symptoms mentioned above require special attention: trigeminal neuralgia and the MS hug. Trigeminal neuralgia has to be one of the worst symptoms that people with multiple sclerosis experience. A couple of readers have written to me about this symptom and said that there were no words to describe the intensity of their pain. Also called *tic douloureux* (French for "painful twitch"), it can be described as an intense, sharp pain, like an electrical jolt, occurring in the lower part of the face, which is often triggered by chewing, drinking, or brushing one's teeth. Usually the most intense pain is short-lived, lasting a couple seconds or minutes, but can result in a more constant burning or aching. The MS hug is the result of tiny muscles between each rib (intercostal muscles) going into spasm. It can be anywhere on the torso (either localized or encircling the body), come in waves or just be constant, and is described as sharp, dull, or burning pain, or a crushing or constricting sensation of intense pressure. Some people experience difficult or painful breathing, which may be so severe that it can be perceived as a heart attack or panic attack.

Fight Back Against Pain

The very first things that you must do to get relief from your pain are to speak up and insist that you be heard and taken seriously. If your doctor insists that MS is painless, consider getting a second opinion or switching doctors altogether. MS *is* painful and the last thing any of us needs is the additional trauma of being made to feel silly or wrong for seeking help for this symptom by the doctor that we are looking to for help.

That said, there are different medications for the different types of pain, depending on the cause and severity. Carbamazepine (Tegretol) or phenytoin (Dilantin) may be effective against trigeminal neuralgia.

Severe burning (dysesthesia) or the MS hug might be effectively treated with gabapentin (Neurontin) or amitriptyline (Elavil). To treat neuropathic pain, some docs are having success with duloxetine hydrochloride (Cymbalta), an antidepressant also used to treat pain associated with diabetic peripheral neuropathy; and pregabalin (Lyrica), a drug for the treatment of neuropathic pain associated with diabetes, fibromyalgia, and certain types of seizures.

Secondary pain caused by awkward gaits or long periods of immobility can often be relieved by over-the-counter non-steroidal anti-inflammatory drugs (NSAIDs), such as acetaminophen (Tylenol) and ibuprofen (Advil or Motrin).

In your quest for pain relief, some CAM modalities might be worth exploring. In some situations, massage, hot compresses or heating pads, biofeedback, or acupuncture can help. If your doctor is willing to experiment, low dose naltrexone is reported by many of its fans to help. Many people claim that marijuana is the only thing that helps their pain.

Numbness and Tingling

In many ways, this is the "MSiest-feeling" symptom that I grapple with. Medical writers and physicians often refer to MS-related numbness and tingling as "only an annoyance," "not disabling," or a "benign" symptom, which informs me that the person has probably never experienced this symptom. In my case, the itching, burning, and tingling have been a minor form of physical and emotional torture—it has interfered with my walking to some degree, but worse than that was the psychological distress caused by its constant presence.

What Paresthesia Feels Like and How It Can Affect Your Life

Most commonly referred to as "numbness" or "tingling," this is one of the MS symptoms that most people initially seek help for, as it is so common in MS and it is immediately clear that it has neurological origins, as opposed to more vague symptoms, such as constipation or fatigue. It feels like numbness, pins and needles, burning, severe itchiness, tingling, buzzing, or vibrating sensations. Paresthesia can be transient or last for a long time. The numbness and tingling can vary in intensity and can come at different times of the day. It can feel like waves of sensation or steady throbbing. In other words, everyone has his or her own special form of paresthesia.

The Real World

The words "numbness and tingling" do not do this symptom justice. Those words do not evoke empathy from doctors, friends, or family. I prefer to say "paresthesia," as in, "My paresthesia is pure torture today," when I want people to pay attention to my complaints.

In my opinion, the impact of pareesthesia is quite underestimated. This burning, tingling, itchy numbness can cause many problems for people with MS. When present in the feet, it can interfere with walking, if one is afraid or hesitant to take a step due to pain, sensory ataxia, and interference with proprioception. Numbness in hands and fingers makes writing, buttoning clothes, tying shoes, and holding small objects next to impossible, and it makes using knives downright dangerous.

Know Your Stuff

Sensory ataxia is a lack of coordination caused by numbness in the feet.

Proprioception, often referred to as the "sixth sense," is the awareness of where our bodies are and how they are positioned in our environment. Loss of proprioception is common in MS, as it is based on constant sensory input from the joints and muscles, which can be slowed down by demyelination. For fun, test your proprioception by holding your arms straight out in front of you and closing your eyes. Swaying while you do this is known as "Romberg's sign" and indicates loss of proprioception.

Paresthesias steal the joy one can get from some of life's great pleasures—sex, good conversations, food, and sleep. Unpleasant sensations in the genital region can make sex almost impossible—certainly enjoyable sex is out of the question. If the tongue is numb, this leads to problems speaking, such as dysarthria, the slurring of words. A numb tongue may also make it difficult to detect the temperature of food. Paresthesias tend to be worse at night and may significantly disturb sleep.

Allodynia is a particular type of paresthesia that happens in response to a stimulus, such as being touched by someone or having clothing or bed sheets brush against the skin. I have read sad accounts of people who are unable to tolerate a hug from their spouse or children because of the pain. Allodynia is stimulus-dependent and only lasts as long as the stimulus is present. The good news is that it is usually a short-term problem.

Fight Back Against Paresthesia

I hate to tell you this, but this is one of those situations where doctors can do very little to help us. In some cases, docs might try a med such as gabapentin (Neurontin) or amitriptyline (Elavil), but these have side effects, including fatigue, and only limited success against numbness and tingling in the extremities has been demonstrated. If you are being tortured by their symptom, your doc might prescribe Solu-Medrol, especially if an MRI confirms that you are having a relapse.

I would start my quest for relief with complementary and alternative approaches, namely creative visualization, biofeedback, and meditation. I know that guided meditation using an audio program has helped me find relief in the past. Low dose naltrexone has also brought relief to some people. Of course, staying cool in hot weather can also help prevent this symptom from getting worse in the heat.

Optic Neuritis and Other Vision Problems

"Okay," I thought to myself as I woke up enough to realize that I was blind in one eye during a research trip to Moscow, "this will be okay." The night before I thought I had a smudge on my contact lens, but now there was a silver fog that completely blocked the middle of my field of vision. I knew that I had MS and I pretty well guessed that this was optic neuritis, so I wasn't overly freaked out about what it might be. Rather, in the two days it took me to get home, my anxiety stemmed from being unable to see in unfamiliar surroundings and it was becoming incredibly painful to move my eyes. A course of Solu-Medrol banished the blindness and the pain, and my vision continued to improve over a couple of months. I will say that I still can't focus well with that eye well and colors seem drab and faded, especially when I get even slightly overheated.

Between 30 to 40 percent of people with MS will have an episode of optic neuritis at some point. Optic neuritis is often the first symptom that leads to a diagnosis of MS. In fact, between 50 and 60 percent of people who have an isolated episode of optic neuritis go on to develop MS. Optic neuritis in MS is caused by a lesion and the related inflammation on the optic nerve.

Don't Panic

We rely on our vision and any change in our eyesight can be terrifying. Remember that the most common MS-related vision problems are (usually) temporary.

What MS-Related Vision Problems Feel Like and How They Can Affect Your Life

Optic neuritis is pretty unmistakable. In most cases, it only occurs in one eye and it is painful, especially when moving the eyes side to side—but the pain usually subsides after a couple of days. It worsens fairly rapidly, with peak vision loss occurring within 24 to 48 hours of onset. It affects the vision in different ways, including: blurring, reduced light, absence of color, flashes of light when the eyes are moved (called phosphenes), and a "blank spot" in the middle of the eye (called a scotoma).

It's pretty rare for optic neuritis to affect both eyes at once—that is the good news. Nevertheless, during a bout of optic neuritis, vision loss in the affected eye can be quite substantial—even complete blindness is not uncommon. Most people recover quite well from optic neuritis and regain their vision. However, some permanent residual loss of clarity or reduced color perception in the affected eye is common.

Two other vision-associated symptoms of MS are nystagmus and diplopia. Nystagmus is involuntary, rapid repetitive movements of the eyes (jiggling eyes), usually from side to side. For some people, it happens only when they look to the side, in others it can be severe and constant enough to impair vision. Diplopia is a fancy term for "double vision," where one object is seen as two objects.

Fight Back Against Vision Problems

There are no effective symptomatic treatments for optic neuritis, nystagmus, or diplopia, and these usually tend to go away on their own, although corticosteroids (such as Solu-Medrol) are sometimes given to reduce the severity or duration of these symptoms. Over 90% of people begin to recover from optic neuritis on their own within a month without steroid treatment, and it is thought that using Solu-Medrol has no effect (positive or negative) on long-term vision. After recovery from a bout of optic neuritis, staying cool will prevent Uthoff's phenomenon, a loss of vision in the heat or during an infection that causes a fever. Vision loss that is a result of any of these problems is not typically helped by glasses. In the case of diplopia, covering one eye with a patch eliminates the double vision and is useful for driving or other necessary tasks, but is not recommended for long periods.

Tremor

It is estimated that up to 75 percent of people with MS experience tremor at some point, usually developing after people have had MS for at least five years. I had several episodes of intention tremor in my hands that would come for a couple of weeks. One such experience occurred when I was working in a research laboratory, preventing me from performing necessary small movements (such as transferring liquid between miniscule vials using a pipette) to carry out experiments. As I was on the verge of quitting, the tremor vanished. These days I might notice an occasional slight tremor when I am trying to use tweezers or mince garlic, but for the most part, it doesn't interfere with anything I am trying to do. My husband and other people, however, have noticed tremor in my head or hands that I am completely unaware of.

Get Help

Not being able to write or open something because of shaky hands can be embarrassing. People notice and become concerned. Be prepared to explain your MS and ask for help.

What MS-Related Tremor Feels Like and How It Can Affect Your Life

Tremors are involuntary muscular contractions that result in a rhythmic back-and-forth movement of a specific body part, usually hands. The two types of tremor associated with multiple sclerosis are intention tremor and postural tremor. Intention tremor occurs when you reach for something and your hand starts shaking. The closer you get to your target or the smaller and more precise the movement required, the more your hand or arm will shake. Postural tremor is shaking that occurs while you are sitting or standing and your muscles are trying to hold parts of your body still against the force of gravity. In rare cases, people experience tremor of the jaw, lips or tongue, which may affect their ability to speak clearly.

For most of us who experience tremor, it is annoying and can be embarrassing. You can go through periods where you are unable to perform precise movements. A tiny percentage of people, however, may experience tremor so severe that it becomes impossible to perform necessary tasks like eating, drinking, or getting dressed.

Fight Back Against Tremor

Unfortunately, there is not much a doctor can do to help MS-related tremor in terms of prescribing medications. A careful review of current medications, however, may reveal that another drug that you are taking to manage a different symptom may be contributing to your tremor, in which case it might be possible to switch this drug.

Some people claim that relaxation and stress-reducing techniques, such as meditation and biofeedback, have helped lessen their tremor. I know that, in my case, like most of my other symptoms, my tremor is worse when I am stressed out, hot, or tired—cooling down and calming down can often make it manageable enough so that I can get the job at hand done (or at least not get as upset when I can't close the safety pin or mince garlic as finely as I would like to).

If tremor interferes with your daily life, occupational therapists can help immensely by problem-solving routine tasks and introducing new ways of doing things or various nifty devices, gadgets, and workarounds to make life easier.

Sexual Dysfunction

In my case, a healthy, vigorous libido is a sign that I am feeling great physically and emotionally. The problem is that, usually, I am feeling less than great and my sex drive is often nowhere to be found, scared away by fatigue, weird numbness in my pelvis, the pain of the MS hug, and the inability to concentrate because of constant "buzzy thoughts" related to cognitive dysfunction. When just getting through the day and taking care of basic needs requires all the attention and effort we can muster, it is easy to put sex in the category of things that are nonessential. What a mistake that is. A good sex life is a critical component of wellbeing. Not only does sex do nice things on a physical level, such as release lovely endorphins and distract us from our symptoms through fun sensations, it also plays a crucial role in reminding us that we are more than our MS and our spouses or partners are more than caretakers.

Make It Better

Be bold in working to fix sexual dysfunction—ask for help. You might be surprised how much a doctor or therapist can help improve your sex life, and you may find out just how much you were missing.

What MS-Related Sexual Dysfunction Feels Like and How It Can Affect Your Life

Women with MS may experience a range of sexual problems, including: vaginal dryness, reduced sensation or exaggerated sensitivity in the vaginal area, difficulty with the movements and positions involved in sex due to pain or muscle spasms, loss of libido (interest in sex), and difficulty having orgasms. Men with MS may experience the following sexual problems: reduced sensitivity in the penis, difficulty getting or keeping an erection (erectile dysfunction), difficulty with ejaculation (dry orgasm), loss of libido, or difficulty with the movements or positions involved in sex.

For both sexes, sexual dysfunction can harm or even destroy a relationship, especially if there is not good communication.

Fight Back Against Sexual Dysfunction

Communication with your partner is by far the most important component of the solution to sexual dysfunction, and often the most difficult. Men and women with MS are probably already experiencing some degree of anger, embarrassment, fatigue, and grief as a result of the changes in their bodies, so bringing up the subject of sexual dysfunction may be frightening. It is crucial to seek help from your doctor, even though this may be uncomfortable. Many treatments exist for both female and male sexual dysfunction, but your doctor cannot help you with your sexual concerns unless you mention them. Some sexual problems are actually medication side effects, which can be handled by adjusting medications that you are already taking or changing the time of day that you take medications.

Medical approaches for men experiencing erectile dysfunction can include medications such as Viagra and Cialis, which work in about 50 percent of men with MS. There are also medications that can be injected into the base of the penis to produce an erection and devices that can be surgically inserted into the penis to assist with erections. Women can often get help from vaginal lubricants or vibrators, and some medications, such as Viagra, work to help women with arousal. Both sexes may benefit from muscle relaxants and pain medications to help spasms and pain that may interfere with sex.

Try different sexual positions, as varying your usual "routine" may relieve some sexual problems, especially if they are related to other MS symptoms, such as pain, weakness or spasticity. Try to have sex when you are feeling your best, even if this does not correspond to the usual timing of sex. Expanding your concept of sex beyond orgasms to include hugging, kissing, and other forms of contact, will keep the intimacy alive. Don't forget that masturbation (solo or with a partner) is part of a normal, healthy sex life.

Vertigo

Vertigo is a fairly common symptom of multiple sclerosis, occurring in about 20% of people with MS at some point. It is an acute, uncomfortable sensation, making those of us who are already a little unsteady feel even more nervous about moving around. Fortunately, it is not a permanent symptom, and may not even indicate a new lesion or inflammation, as vertigo can have non-MS causes. Though it can be caused by lesions in the cerebellum or the nerves that control the vestibular functions of the ear in the brain stem, it appears that a very common cause in people with MS is something called benign paroxysmal positioning vertigo, rather than demyelination, and is in no way related to MS.

Vertigo can also be made worse by some of the drugs prescribed for MS symptoms, such as tricyclic antidepressants (such as Elavil) for neuropathic pain or Baclofen for spasticity, as these drugs can cause dizziness. Lastly, vertigo can be caused by infections, such as the flu.

What Vertigo Feels Like and How It Can Affect Your Life

Vertigo is a sensation of spinning, whether it feels like you are spinning or your surroundings are rotating around you. Think back to when you were a child and spun around and around, then stopped— that's pretty much the sensation of vertigo. It can feel like the ground is suddenly rushing upwards, or that the room is moving continuously or only seems to rotate part of the way, return to normal, and rotate partway again. Vertigo episodes rarely last for a long time, but they can recur for weeks, going away gradually.

> ### Know Your Stuff
>
> In the interest of precision, there is a difference between vertigo and dizziness, both of which are symptoms of MS. Vertigo is a sensation that either yourself or your surroundings are spinning, while dizziness means that you feel faint or lightheaded (like you stood up too fast).

Vertigo can cause people to be very nervous about going out, so they limit their activities, as they are afraid of having an attack. It can be a very powerful feeling of movement and can cause nausea or vomiting. At its worst, it can cause difficulty standing or walking and even lead to falls.

Fight Back Against Vertigo

The first thing that you can do about vertigo is to see an otolaryngologist (aka an ear, nose and throat specialist). An even better choice would be an otoneurologist or a neurotologist, who are specialists in both matters of the inner ear and neurology. It is important to find someone who can untangle MS from vertigo and find the true cause of the symptom, as some cases can be treated without medications, preventing unnecessary MRI scans and potentially fatigue-causing drugs.

Paroxysmal Symptoms

Paroxysmal symptoms come on suddenly, bother us for a short time (seconds or minutes), and then disappear as suddenly as they came. Whether it is an episode of double vision or a prickly feeling on my face, these moments usually lead me to wonder a number of things: Is this a relapse? How bad is this going to get? Does this mean my MS is progressing?

Don't Panic

No need to freak out (immediately) when a symptom flares up— it doesn't necessarily mean a relapse or disease progression, it could be a paroxysmal symptom, especially if it comes and goes and lasts for less than 24 hours.

These symptoms do not mean that you are having a relapse. The good news is that these symptoms are probably just due to a transmission of nerve impulses across sites where they do not normally occur and where there has been previous damage. This phenomenon can be caused by some sort of stimulation, such as irritating clothing or movement. Interestingly, people often experience paroxysmal symptoms having not even been aware that they had a corresponding lesion in the past.

What Paroxysmal Symptoms Feel Like and How They Can Affect Your Life

The bad news is that paroxysmal symptoms tend to recur; they can happen several times a day, or on a daily or weekly basis. Almost any symptom of MS can appear and disappear in this manner, but the most common ones to behave this way include: diplopia (double vision); parasthesia (numbness and tingling); ataxia (sudden unsteadiness or lack of coordination); pain (including trigeminal neuralgia and l'Hermitte's sign); muscle weakness; severe itchiness; seizures; and dysarthria (speech disorder in which pronunciation is unclear, due to slurring, volume of voice, or strange speech rhythms, but the meaning of what is said is normal). Seizures in MS are considered by many to be paroxysmal symptoms, and are usually tonic-clonic (sometimes called "grand mal") or simple or complex partial seizures, which do not cause a loss of consciousness, but awareness and responsiveness is altered to different degrees. Akinesia is a particularly striking phenomenon of being unable to move, often described as "freezing in place," which can take the form of full temporary paralysis, or mean that the person can only move slowly or with extreme difficulty.

Although usually only lasting for seconds at a time, different symptoms can be very painful (trigeminal neuralgia or itching), alarming (seizures or akinesia), or socially problematic (dysarthria). People may stop socializing or quit work or school for fear that they might have a seizure or other symptom while in a public place. Restrictions may be put on driving until seizures are brought under control. Some medications for paroxysmal symptoms may make people drowsy, contribute to MS-related fatigue, and may impair functionality at dosages necessary to control the symptoms. As with many other MS symptoms and strategies to manage them, doctors and their patients have to work together to find the right medications and optimal dosages to provide relief from symptoms without unbearable side effects.

Fight Back Against Paroxysmal Symptoms

The good news is that paroxysmal symptoms tend to respond well to low doses of anticonvulsants. Often, when they are treated, they go away and don't come back. You can also find comfort in the fact that these symptoms do *not* signal a relapse—for whatever that is worth.

Uncontrollable Laughing and Crying

Involuntary emotional expression disorder (IEED), also known as pseudobulbar affect, is characterized by outbursts of crying or laughter, but without corresponding emotions behind these outbursts. It is referred to by some as "emotional incontinence," which perhaps is not the most charming description, but pretty accurately sums up the phenomenon.

What IEED Feels Like and How It Can Affect Your Life

In order to begin to understand what the experience of this symptom may be like, put yourself in a couple of imaginary situations. Imagine if, without warning, you suddenly started weeping during a business meeting, in the grocery store, or at a dinner party where you didn't know many people. Perhaps even more upsetting might be if you began laughing hysterically at an inappropriate time, like during a funeral or wedding.

Make It Better

Though rare, keep IEED in mind if you experience episodes of laughing or crying that seem out of sync with your emotions at the time. Also, it might take a long time for someone to figure out that your laughing or crying is an MS symptom and it may be a good idea to explain IEED to them to avoid hurt feelings and minimize awkwardness.

IEED is often missed by physicians treating people with MS, because they assume the crying outbursts are a manifestation of depression, an extremely common symptom of MS. Indeed, many people with IEED are confused, frustrated and angry about the problem and this further leads to difficulty communicating with their doctors about it.

Fight Back Against IEED

Help your doctor make the right diagnosis and differentiate your situation from depression by: telling him if your emotions don't match your reactions; you don't have thoughts of helplessness, hopelessness or guilt; you are not experiencing problems or changes in sleep or appetite; and your crying (or laughing) comes on and ends very suddenly.

Prepare a little speech to explain a little bit about IEED to your loved ones or people that you work with. This way, when you do find yourself laughing or crying, you will have something ready to say that is not clouded by embarrassment, frustration, or anger. This can greatly reduce stress.

In the past, IEED was treated with low doses of tricyclic antidepressants, such as amitriptyline and nortriptyline, with limited success. Selective serotonin reuptake inhibitors (SSRIs) are also used and help some people. The most promise, however, is being shown by a new drug that is being developed specifically for IEED and diabetic peripheral neuropathy by Avanir Pharmaceuticals, called Zenvia (dextromethorphan hydrobromide/quinidine sulfate).

Problems Swallowing

Here's another often-overlooked symptom of MS that I have added to my personal collection—between 30 and 40 percent of people with MS experience swallowing problems at some time. Also referred to as "dysphagia," swallowing problems are typically caused by lesions on the nerves along the pathways that coordinate muscles used in swallowing or the brainstem. Dysphagia can also be caused or made worse by a lack of saliva or dry mouth, which can be a result of different medications used to control symptoms.

I'll admit that I wasn't that excited to find out that dysphagia is yet another MS symptom that I might have, much less how common it is. This does, however, explain how frequently I've coughed so hard when attempting to swallow a pill that I have nearly passed out. I also have learned the hard way that I should not have dinner with people that I find extremely amusing, as laughing and eating are a very dangerous mix for me, causing choking and sputtering and all sorts of undignified efforts to catch my breath.

What Swallowing Problems Feel Like and How They Can Affect Your Life

Many people with MS-related swallowing problems are not aware of this symptom besides experiencing the occasional coughing fit after something "goes down the wrong way." Dysphagia, though, includes many different impediments with the swallowing process—some of which don't seem directly related to swallowing food or liquids—including difficulty chewing, food sticking in the throat, the feeling that it is hard to swallow food or move it to the back of the mouth, coughing while eating or immediately afterward, producing excessive saliva or drooling, choking, vomiting food back up, and speaking in a weak or soft voice. Aspiration, meaning that food or liquid is going down the windpipe into the lungs, can also occur.

Make It Better

Most people eat much too fast—use dysphagia as a reason to slow down and enjoy your food more. If it becomes severe, seek help through your MS doc.

For the most part, those of us with a "touch of dysphagia" can pretty much go about our business, as long as we are aware of the situation and pay attention to eating and drinking slowly and mindfully. Dysphagia can become so severe, however, that people become dehydrated or malnourished. If the tips for managing swallowing difficulties don't work, it may be necessary to use a feeding tube.

Food or liquids that end up in the lungs can cause aspiration pneumonia. This is a particularly dangerous lung infection, especially in people that are not very mobile, and is actually a leading cause of death in people with MS.

Fight Back Against Swallowing Problems

The first things to try are the things that your mother would want you to do anyway: Sit up straight. Don't talk with your mouth full. Slow down when you eat. Take smaller bites. Some people find relief when they add thickener to liquids or avoid hard, crunchy foods. Alternating liquids and solids may also help keep the food moving in the right direction. If you are feeling very "MSy" with very pronounced symptoms at a certain time, be extra careful when you eat. Tuck your chin in toward your chest slightly while swallowing, as moving your chin in one-half inch closes off the airways, preventing food and liquid from going into your respiratory passages.

If you are still experiencing problems, you can get referred to a speech and language pathologist, who will watch you eat and drink and may perform a test called a videofloroscopy, which is an x-ray video of the swallowing process. That will help them determine how to instruct you to avoid problems. If you have many chest infections, make sure the cause is investigated so that you can avoid complications in the future.

Important note: Everyone in your household, including yourself, should learn the Heimlich maneuver. The Heimlich maneuver is a preventive emergency measure to use to dislodge food when someone is choking, which you can also perform on yourself. Learn the Heimlich maneuver at www.heimlichinstitute.org. It's just a good idea.

Respiratory Dysfunction

I'm always frightened by the first tickle of a sore throat each winter, as it is often the harbinger of a minor infection that will become a terrible cough that lasts for months. While I haven't had my lung function measured, I am fairly sure that I would test pretty low on pulmonary function tests, as would most MSers.

What Respiratory Dysfunction Feels Like and How It Can Affect Your Life

Fortunately, for most of us, these problems are not noticeable or do not impede us in any significant way. MS-related respiratory problems can take several forms, including: shortness of breath, coughing, hiccupping, frequent sighing, or difficulty breathing deeply. The resulting sensations of not getting enough air can be described as the feeling of having a heavy weight on the chest or trying to breathe with a heavy blanket over your nose and mouth.

Make It Better

It's nearly impossible at times to know if your respiratory symptoms are because of MS, allergies, or a cold. You can help yourself by creating a healthy environment for your lungs and avoiding things like cigarette smoke and potential allergens, while exercising your lungs daily with cardio workouts or specific "lung training."

First of all, you can eliminate the "worst case scenario" from your head. It is extremely rare that MS-related breathing difficulties ever become so severe that they are life-threatening or that people require breathing assistance, such as breathing tubes or supplemental oxygen.

However, even fairly mild breathing problems can cause severe fatigue. I have my suspicions that many MSers (myself included) suffer from this type of "subclinical" respiratory problem. I also suspect that MS-related respiratory dysfunction makes it more difficult to shake upper respiratory infections, which often turn into bronchitis. The feeling that you can't get enough air can lead to panic attacks and severe anxiety.

Fight Back Against Respiratory Dysfunction

It appears that breathing exercises to prevent respiratory complications during later stages of MS (as well as improve overall respiratory function) are successful at improving breathing capacity. One device that is showing promise in helping people with MS "train" their lungs is called PowerLung (www.powerlung.com), a handheld device that can be used at home and costs under 100 dollars. In addition, regular cardiovascular exercise can improve a person's aerobic capacity, which is the amount of oxygen your body can use during exercise. This can help with fatigue.

Constipation

There are two crucial components to regular bowel movements: the stool must keep moving through the intestines and there must be enough water in the stool. Constipation in people with MS can be caused by a combination of many factors that interfere with these things. Neurological damage can impact the voluntary and involuntary sensations and movements that keep stool moving, and restricted physical activity also affects motility. Many of us also limit fluid intake in (misguided) attempts to counter bladder-related symptoms, causing our stools to be hard and dry. Constipation can also be caused by certain medications that we take for symptoms, such as antispasticity drugs, antidepressants, and drugs for bladder dysfunction.

What Constipation Feels Like and How It Can Affect Your Life

Pretty much everyone has been constipated and knows what it feels like. However, there is a more precise definition than just "I can't go," which includes having two or fewer bowel movements per week, feeling like you have not eliminated the entire bowel movement at least 25% of the time, straining to have a bowel movement at least 25% of the time, and having a lumpy or hard stool at least 25% of the time.

> **Make It Better**
>
> Managing constipation is one of the more straightforward MS symptoms to improve with things you can do on your own. Follow the suggestions here and see if you can't get control over this symptom.

In most cases, constipation ranges from mildly annoying to pretty substantially uncomfortable. In some cases, it can act as a "noxious stimulus" for spasticity, dysesthesia, or the MS hug. Constipation that is not managed can result in fecal impaction, which happens when constipation is so severe that the entire rectum becomes filled with a large, hard ball of stool. In these cases, manual disimpaction is needed, meaning that a doctor or a nurse removes the blockage manually.

Fight Back Against Constipation

In many cases, constipation can be successfully addressed by drinking more caffeine-free fluids (caffeine is a diuretic, so can contribute to the problem), moving around more, and eating a diet higher in fiber. In line with more "natural" approaches, you can add in ground psyllium or flaxseeds to your diet by mixing a tablespoon into a large glass of water or fruit juice and following it with another glass of water. You can also get things moving with prune juice or other types of juices (some claim that pear juice, beet juice or aloe vera juice work wonders). Stool softeners can also be taken for short periods. If these things don't work to give you the relief that you need, you should speak to your doctor about next steps. Although laxatives (both herbal and chemical) can work wonders, they should be used with caution, as should enemas, and neither should be used for more than one week unless your doctor tells you it is okay.

Speech Difficulties

I hate this one, I hate it. To me, it is pure torture to hear the MS in my voice as I am talking to someone. In the middle of a conversation, usually a very important one, I can tell that my speaking cadence and rhythm are bizarre. Often, this is taken even further by my tongue tripping over syllables, slurring parts of words as I try to push them out. The result, to my ears, sounds like a toddler speaking English as a foreign language while frantically trying to communicate something of great urgency.

What Speech Difficulties Feel Like and How They Can Affect Your Life

The speech of someone with MS can be affected by dysarthria and dysphonia, which are speech disorders in which the pronunciation is unclear, but the meaning of what is said is normal. Dysarthria usually results from lesions in the cerebellum and can affect the pitch of the voice, resonance and articulation (how clearly and precisely words are pronounced). Scanning speech is a form of dysarthria that causes people to speak in slow or strange rhythms, where syllables of words are separated by long pauses. Dysphonia is an impairment of the voice, which can include hoarseness, raspy speech, or a change in pitch when the person tries to talk. Dysphonia in people with MS usually manifests as trouble controlling the volume of speech, meaning people end up speaking too softly to be heard or more loudly than is appropriate.

Know Your Stuff

Read this section carefully. Take the time to remember the different ways MS can impact your speech so that you can evaluate what is happening, lessening frustration and embarrassment. These types of confusion and communication problems can be devastating, but more so if you forget that MS is the cause and not some new neurological or social problem.

Both dysarthria and dysphonia should be differentiated from dysphasia, a problem understanding or communicating using spoken or written words, which is also a symptom of MS. Cognitive dysfunction can lead to dysphasia-related word-finding difficulties, which also affects the overall fluidity of speech and ease of communication.

Only a very tiny percentage of people with MS will be rendered unable to speak. However, if this happens, there are assistive devices available to help with communication, including high-tech options like devices with simulated voices and low-tech options like hand-held cards.

Fight Back Against Speech Difficulties

As bad as it sounds to my ears, I probably have a pretty mild case of both dysarthria and dysphonia, which comes and goes and is worse when I am hot or tired. I find that cooling down and slowing down help a great deal. When I feel that I am having this problem, I work on keeping sentences short and simple and trying to stay calm and relaxed. If simple measures do not adequately control your problem or if your speech disorders are impacting your work or other aspects of your life, a speech/language pathologist is a professional who can evaluate the situation. He or she can work with you and give you exercises to do on your own to improve your enunciation and overall rhythm of speech.

How to Talk to Your Doctor About Your Symptoms

When we visit our doctor, the most helpful information he or she has comes from the details that we can give about our symptoms and our experiences living with these symptoms. This is especially true of the symptoms that we feel, such as pain or fatigue, as opposed to those that can be measured objectively, such as walking speed or range of motion. In most cases, there are treatments that can help, but the doctor must be able to determine the most likely cause of the symptom and how much it is affecting your life before deciding which therapy to try and how aggressive to be in a symptom management approach.

Here are some questions that you doctor might ask about a symptom—let's use fatigue as our example of how we might answer the questions using the most helpful level of detail and relevance:

How long does the fatigue typically last? The doc will be trying to determine if the fatigue is paroxysmal (meaning it comes on suddenly and sporadically, then leaves just as suddenly) or chronic (meaning it comes on more slowly and sticks around for a long time before slowly fading away or lessening). The first type of fatigue could be due to an environmental factor, such as heat intolerance, which could be alleviated by trying simple things to avoid that situation.

How often does it happen? Try to be precise in your answer to this and include information from the question above about duration. For instance, has the fatigue occurred every day in the morning for the past two weeks and lasted until you took a nap? Or does the fatigue seem to come every couple of months for the past year and stay for 3 days straight each time until slowly resolving?

Take Charge

Details, details, details. Make sure you have all the information possible about your symptom. This will guide choices about medications and therapies. Accuracy is critical here to avoid choosing the wrong approach and missing an opportunity to make things better.

When is it the worst? Do you feel worse when you first wake up or does the fatigue seem to worsen as the day wears on? Does it hit you suddenly every day, an hour after taking your morning medication or 30 minutes before lunch, or does the onset seem more random?

How would you describe your fatigue? You can get descriptive here and give answers such as, "It feels like I am moving through quicksand" or "It feels like I have a hangover that doesn't get better." Answer with as much detail as you can, avoiding simple, obvious answers such as "I get tired."

How intense is your fatigue? See if you can rate your fatigue on a scale of 1 to 10, with "1" being a very slight tiredness and "10" being the most exhausted you have ever been (or worse). When my fatigue is in "full bloom," I wake up with a dreadful tiredness (about a 7.5) that gets punctuated with 15-minute spells of immobility (pretty much a "10"), to the point that I have to put my head down wherever I am.

Does the fatigue affect your daily activities? Has the fatigue kept you home from work? Have you not kept up with your usual chores around the house because of the fatigue? Have there been any times that you were supposed to spend time with friends and family that you canceled, or have there been times when you did not engage in your favorite hobbies because of the fatigue? Has your fatigue affected your sex life? I know that there were a couple of times when I was afraid to be the only one watching my toddler twins because of the intensity of the fatigue. That was when I was compelled to ask my doc for medication.

Have you noticed that anything makes it feel better or worse? Think hard about this one. Does the fatigue get more intense after you have been in the sun? Is the fatigue worsened by stress? Stress and fatigue can make each other worse in a vicious cycle, where a little fatigue causes worry that it will get worse, and, in turn, this stress actually does have a negative effect on the fatigue.

How effective are your current fatigue medications? Talk about all medications and remedies that you have tried for your fatigue, including over-the-counter drugs and any illegal drugs you may have tried. It is important to tell all of these things to the doctor, even if you are pretty sure he will think it was not such a fabulous idea to use these things. Rate their effects on a scale of 1 to 10—"1" being that you detected no effect at all and "10" meaning that your fatigue quickly and completely disappeared. Don't forget to mention caffeine use if you have been drinking copious amounts of coffee to try to combat the fatigue. Also mention any other things you may have tried, including acupuncture, massage, biofeedback, or other complementary and alternative methods.

Again, I used fatigue in the above example to illustrate the kinds of details doctors want to know about symptoms. Approach the discussion of any symptom (pain, depression, tremor, sensory disturbances, sexual dysfunction) with your doctor in a constructive manner, using a similar level of detail and information. Remember, the doctor is relying on us to provide pertinent information about a symptom so that he can figure out the best course of action. Even if there are further tests that can be run in the case of particular symptoms, a good account of your experiences may guide the decision about the best way to investigate further.

The Bottom Line

Because there are over 80 symptoms associated with multiple sclerosis, this chapter is meant to serve as an overview of some of the most common ones. When you think you might be experiencing a new symptom, check in with yourself and truly evaluate what is happening physically, rather than allowing emotions of fear or denial to take over. Discuss your symptoms with your doctor in a thorough, thoughtful way and make sure that you are listened to. It is one thing if there simply are no good solutions for managing a symptom, but another if your doctor denies that you are having a certain symptom in the first place or tells you that your discomfort is entirely a result of stress. There are many, many ways to find relief from symptoms and your doctor should help you think outside the box, giving you tips to try at home and recommending (or at least answering your questions about) complementary and alternative therapies if there are some that might have a chance at helping you.

Be assertive. Get the help you need. Keep trying. Don't give up. Attain the highest quality of life that you can.

4

Make Your Doctor Work for You

The doc that gave me my MS diagnosis was big into theatrics and really crappy in terms of bedside manner. He whipped my MRI films into the lightbox with a flourish and pointed out my lesions by saying, "Look at this one! Boy, a couple millimeters to the left and you would be incontinent." I swear, I think he actually let out a little giggle. I don't know, it just seems like an extra and unnecessary blow to be told you have a chronic illness by someone that you have little confidence in (and kind of hate).

The fact remains that those of us with MS clearly require medical care. There are diagnostic tests to undergo, treatment options to pursue, symptoms to manage, and many other things that bring us into contact with doctors, nurses, and the medical system. Whereas a broken arm or strep throat can be adequately taken care of by someone you see once or twice and have no rapport with, MS is different—it is incurable. We will have MS for the rest of our lives, we therefore will need medical care for our MS for the rest of our lives.

The Real World

MS is not curable. That means you'll be seeing some doctor for your MS for the rest of your life. Put in the time to make sure your doctor is the right one for you.

It is crucial that we rise to the challenge of actively participating in our medical care. However, medical situations have an interesting effect on many of us. We might be powerhouses in the boardroom, people who do not hesitate to challenge our friends if we suspect an injustice, and/or parents who stop at nothing to ensure that we are getting the best for our children; however, when it comes to our own medical care, we tend to turn over more of ourselves to the doctor, participating less in medical decisions about our bodies than in discussions with waiters about how our meal is prepared.

In order to be involved in our medical care in a beneficial way, we need to get the following things in place: the right doctor for us, productive interactions with our doctors, the confidence and freedom to seek second opinions, and control over our medical information.

Helping You is Your Doctor's Job

I am not one of those angry patients who distrusts and reviles physicians. I love the doctors that I have chosen to stay with as a patient, but it has been a process getting here. From the comments I get from my readers, I can tell that many people have relationships with their doctors that are still a "work in progress," or that need to end altogether, including the following remarks:

> "I always feel worse after visiting my neurologist—he makes me feel like an idiot."

> "Of course, my doctor went to medical school and knows all the fancy words, but he doesn't have MS, and I do. It seems like that would give me a little credibility when I tell him about symptoms that I am feeling. Instead, if it is not in a book, he tells me that I am not feeling it. Just last week, my doctor told me that MS is painless after I told him that my feet were tingling so badly that they hurt like crazy."

> "I feel confused when I go to the doctor. I leave with half my questions unanswered and often don't even understand what he told me about my symptoms or how he is going to treat them."

We all have situations where we nod our heads, even when we have no clue what is being said (for me, discussions of stock futures cause this reaction); accept something told to us, even if we know beyond a doubt that it is not true (my 3-year-old daughter often insists that she is really a white kitten); and endure unfulfilling relationships (fill in your own example here, I don't know which of my peeps are reading this). However, our interactions with our doctors should not resemble *any* of those situations. We must strive for comprehension of what we are told about our bodies and our disease, must have confidence in our doctor's expertise and conclusions, and must perceive that our doctor is our partner, looking out for the our best interests.

> ### Take Charge
>
> Your doctor works for *you*. Get your needs met and feel good about the relationship.

Find the Right Doctor for You

Evaluate Your Doc

As I mentioned, the neurologist that gave me my first tentative MS diagnosis was a jerk. I ended up in his office because I had all sorts of funky symptoms that just screamed "neurological" in nature. I was referred to him by a clinic that I went to because I thought my tingly feet and gripping feeling around my ribcage might be due to a pinched nerve or a vitamin deficiency.

Many people with MS have similar stories about how they ended up with the doctor that diagnosed their MS. After all, how many of us correctly identified our symptoms as neurological in nature and happened to know a fabulous neurologist who was accepting new, self-referred patients?

> ### Take Charge
>
> Evaluate your doctor situation: How did you end up with the doctor who is caring for your MS? Did you actively choose this doctor? Are you happy with him or her? What are the pros and cons of your current doc?

When a diagnosis of multiple sclerosis is made, people often feel very emotional and committed to the doctor that helped them figure out what was wrong, as well as overwhelmed and confused. The nature of most cases of MS is that they are unpredictable and act up sporadically, meaning that you may need to see the doctor very frequently for awhile, then six months will go by where there is no need to see him. During these quiet spells it is easy to forget, or at least ignore, negative feelings about your doctor or the care that you are receiving.

Whether you just got diagnosed or you have been with one doctor for a long time, it is a good idea to take a long, hard look at your doctor. After all, you have not married this person or given birth to him or her (in most cases), so deciding that he or she is not the one for you is a relatively simple problem to fix.

Even if your current neurologist is supposed to be the MS king in your area, it is no good if you feel worse than you did when you went in because you were not listened to or taken seriously. Some people, however, expect to feel overwhelmed in a doctor's presence. I think many of us pretty much know how we feel about our current doctor, but it wouldn't hurt to take a look at this list of questions and see how your doc is doing:

Does your doctor spend at least 15 minutes with you?

When you ask about a new drug or the possibility of switching treatment, does your doctor listen, or does he dismiss the idea without giving a reason?

Do you feel like your doctor adequately discusses the important things about new drugs (possible side effects, best results to expect, how long until the medication starts working) or symptoms that you might have (how bad it might get, different treatment options)?

Are you treated with respect by the office staff, the nurses, and the doctor?

When you tell your doctor about a new symptom, does he ever roll his eyes, tell you that what you are feeling is not possible, or say anything else insensitive?

Do you and your doctor actually discuss options for your treatment, or is it more a situation of being told by the doctor what the next steps are?

How comfortable are you (or would you be) discussing a potentially embarrassing or confusing symptom with your doctor?

Do you feel you can call your doctor to ask about side effects of drugs or new symptoms that you have without making an appointment?

What does your gut say? Will this doctor be a good partner for you in the long-term?

I love my current neurologist. He can be kind of rough in his handling of me and my feelings, but I don't mind. It seems a little like tough love, and I guess he figures I can take it. Once, when I presented him with an experimental treatment I wanted him to "score" for me, he told me that he wouldn't get it for me, he thought it was stupid and he was surprised that someone "as smart as me" would even ask (I guess that softened the tirade a little). Despite all this, he does listen carefully, he troubleshoots with me, and he makes the neurology fellows studying under him call me "doctor," despite the fact that I am a PhD, not an MD. He also fought with my insurance company to ensure that I would be approved for in vitro fertilization treatment when it became clear that I couldn't afford the time to try to conceive on my own while delaying treatment for MS. Overall, the most important thing is that my gut tells me that he has my best interests at heart.

The Real World

Remember, living with MS is about more than keeping the MS at bay and annual MRIs. Over time, you may have dozens of symptoms that require treatment. Can you talk about these symptoms with your doctor so that he or she understands what impact they really have on your life?

Know What You Want in a Doctor

When we were shopping for our home, my husband became increasingly frustrated with the details that I was attracted to. "Ooh, look at those pretty daffodils," I would say even before we opened the door, "I love this house." I would also be swayed (both in positive and negative directions) by the current owner's taste in furniture or paint colors. Luckily, the home we ended up with has turned out to be perfect for us, despite the fact that the big selling point for me was a tiny cardinal's nest in a tree by the front door.

Take Charge

You can't find the right doctor if you don't know what you want.

Just as it sounds silly to be swayed by superficial and transient details when choosing a house to buy, it is important that you know what you want in an MS doctor. Sure, a pretty waiting room with current issues of frivolous design and celebrity gossip magazines is always an asset. The relationship will go deeper than that, however, resulting in decisions that you have to adhere to and live with after you leave the office.

Take a couple of minutes and consider the following characteristics of what you might want in a doctor:

Neurologist or general practitioner? I strongly recommend that you see a neurologist for treatment of your MS. A 2008 study in the journal *Neurology* found that approximately 28% of people consult non-neurologists (most of these were primary care physicians) for their MS care.[1] The main finding of the study was that the people who saw non-neurologists might not be getting the best treatment for their MS. It turned out that the people seeing neurologists were significantly more likely to take disease-modifying drugs; attend an outpatient program; and see occupational therapists, urologists, or physical therapists. Interestingly, the people who were seeing non-neurologists tended to have more disability, in that more required wheelchairs or were confined to bed.

Does the doctor specialize in MS? Among neurologists, there are those that specialize only in the treatment of MS, whereas others treat all different kinds of neurological diseases and disorders in addition to MS, such as stroke, Alzheimer's disease, and epilepsy. The MS specialists have seen many more patients with MS and a much broader variety of symptoms, including rare ones. Though it is true that every case of MS is unique, doctors who see "all MS, all the time" are more likely to have seen situations very similar to yours. That will help them to predict what medication might be the most effective for you, what side effects you might experience, and what course your MS might take.

Is the doctor affiliated with an MS clinic? If you are lucky enough to live within a reasonable distance to an MS clinic, you may want to give serious consideration to becoming a patient there. The benefits can be huge. The clinic may participate in a number of clinical trials and be aware of others that may be appropriate for you. Most likely, the MS center has strong relationships with the specialists and therapists that people with MS might need, even in obscure fields, such as neuropsychology, neuroopthamology, psychiatry with experience with MS patients, occupational and physical therapy specializing in MS, and others. In addition, the staff of MS clinics can often answer many of your questions over the phone.

What is the doctor's approach to treating MS? Some neurologists like to leave big decisions, such as which disease-modifying drug to try (or whether to start treatment at all) up to the patient. Others have very definite preferences for certain medications, to the point that they may be referred to as "the Avonex guy" or "that Copaxone doc" and be very reluctant, or even unwilling, to prescribe anything else. Still others interview the patients at length about certain lifestyle factors, their expectations and fears, as well as their history. The doctor will then combine what the patient has told them with their experience with the various drugs in similar cases and make a recommendation based on all of these factors.

In addition, only certain doctors are allowed to prescribe Tysabri, as the facility has to be registered with the TOUCH (stands for TYSABRI Outreach: Unified Commitment to Health) program. This is the monitoring program implemented after the occurrence of Tysabri-related cases of progressive multifocal leukoencephalopathy (PML) in an attempt to catch any potential cases in early stages, as well as prevent them.

The Real World

Learn the backstory to new treatments, especially before insisting that your doc consider them in your case. The situation is usually more complex than you might think.

Doctors also differ in their approach to managing progressive forms of MS. They may just wait until your symptoms bring you in, or they may want to see you quarterly. They may want you to have regular

MRI scans to monitor disease progression, or they may not care about MRIs at all, preferring to rely on clinical findings.

Also, some docs will readily and happily send you to other professionals or therapists to solve a problem or manage a symptom. Others may wait until you ask to be referred. Some doctors take care of managing the integrated care, whereas others simply tell you what kind of specialist you need or give you a phone number and send you on your way. It pays to figure out what the ideal approach is for you—some of us would prefer to be told to go here at this time, while other people like to participate in researching other physicians and setting up their own appointments according to their schedules.

How aggressive do you want your doctor to be in your treatment? Decide if you are the type of person who wants to try the newest or the strongest approach to managing a symptom or bringing a relapse under control. Maybe you prefer a more conservative "wait and see" approach to dealing with your symptoms. There isn't a universal correct answer here, but you should know which strategy you are the most comfortable with and make sure that your doctor is supportive of this route.

What are the doctor's research interests? Researchers are up-to-date on the latest treatments, at least the ones that they are looking at, but often have less time for patient interaction. However, if you have a specific symptom or a rare manifestation of MS that they are interested in, it might be a perfect fit.

Does board certification matter to you? You may wonder what the advantages to having a doctor who is board certified are. Here is the official answer from the website of the American Board of Medical Specialties (ABMS):

> "If your doctor is certified by an ABMS Member Board, it means he or she is dedicated to providing exceptional patient care through a rigorous, voluntary commitment to lifelong learning through board certification and ABMS Maintenance of Certification (MOC). In addition to completing years of schooling, fulfilling residency requirements and passing the exams required to practice medicine in your state, your board certified specialist participates in an ongoing process of continuing education to keep current with the latest advances in medical science and technology in his or her specialty as well as best

practices in patient safety, quality healthcare and creating a responsive patient-focused environment."

Personally, if I found a doctor I liked who wasn't board certified, I would not let that deter me from becoming his patient. I am, however, happy with the knowledge that my neurologist is board certified. As people with MS, we are looking for doctors who are certified in neurology by the American Board of Psychiatry and Neurology. If you are interested in checking out a specific neurologist, you can go to the website of ABMS (www.abms.org) and click on "Is Your Doctor Certified?" You will have to register, but the service is free of charge.

How open is the doctor (and are you) to complementary and alternative medicine (CAM)? Studies show that the majority of us try some form of CAM to try to address our symptoms or slow disease progression at some point after our MS diagnosis. My guess is that most people don't tell their doctors some of the stuff they try, especially if it is really out there. However, many doctors support the use of things like biofeedback, reiki, massage, and reflexology to alleviate symptoms, and most don't object to such noninvasive approaches (they may even be able to recommend practitioners who have experience with MS). Most doctors will tell you that there is no scientific evidence that diet has any effect on MS disease progression but will tell you that by all means you should continue to eat healthier. However, if you are interested in some of the more potent herbal therapies, getting your mercury fillings removed, chelation, bee venom therapy, or any of the more dramatic and potentially dangerous CAM modalities, you should make sure that you feel comfortable sharing these things with your doctor. There are many different ways that supplements or therapies can interact with what your doctor has prescribed for you and it is of utmost importance that he or she is aware of what is going on.

Make It Better

CAM treatments can be great for managing symptoms and just getting through the day. CAM, which includes things like yoga, acupuncture, vitamin supplements, and even prayer, can be just the thing to lift fatigue into the "tolerable" category or get a better night's sleep. You should be able to talk to your doctor about any CAM therapy you are considering or using.

Location and convenience are a consideration. Are you willing to drive a bit farther to see a particular doctor? Does the doctor have appointments in the mornings or evenings? How long does it take to get an appointment? What hospital is the doctor affiliated with? Keep in mind that you may have to get to your doctor during a relapse or time of symptom worsening.

How to Find *Your* Neurologist

Ask a person with MS. Ideally, you would know someone, or know someone who knows someone with MS who *loves* his or her neurologist. I have recommended my doc to about four people—one of them was the daughter of my aunt's best friend, another was my friend's sister-in-law who had just moved to town. I have attended patient education seminars that were actually gigantic advertisements for a specific drug, where the most valuable information was the names of neurologists, physical therapists, and nutritionists being passed around the table as the drug reps droned on up on stage.

If you are fresh out of personal contacts who happen to have MS, support groups can be a great place for referrals. Once you know what you are looking for, you can talk to people at the support group and they will usually be happy to give you recommendations. This is an excellent place to get an honest appraisal of the neurologists in your area.

Take Charge

Spend at least as much time checking out your doctor as you would a babysitter, your daughter's new boyfriend, a new employee, a lawyer, or an accountant. Your doctor is in charge of your MS, you should at least know if she is board certified, how many cases of MS she has treated, and the basics of her plan to manage your MS.

Call your local chapter of the MS society. Your local chapter of the MS Society should have a listing for MS specialists in your area. Give them a call at 1-800-FIGHT-MS (1-800-344-4867) or go to their website to find your local chapter.

Try the Consortium. The Consortium of Multiple Sclerosis Centers is an organization with an inspiring mission: "To be the preeminent professional organization for Multiple Sclerosis healthcare providers and researchers in North America, and a valued partner in the global MS community. Our core purpose is to maximize the ability of MS healthcare providers to impact care of people who are affected by MS, thus improving their quality of life." To help you find one of these doctors who wants to improve your quality of life, the CMSC has a Directory of Centers where you can find a neurologist specializing in MS in your area. The directory is available online at www.mscare.org or the phone number is 201-487-1050. The American Academy of Neurology also has a directory of doctors (go to www.aan.com/go/public and click on "Find a Neurologist"), but no information is given on whether or not they specialize in MS.

Try MSNeuroRatings.com. This is truly the coolest thing for people with MS who are "doc-shopping." It is a very simple forum, focused on only one thing—giving patients a place to rate MS neurologists. Listing doctors from the United States, the United Kingdom, Australia, Canada (and, recently added, Oman), it gives people with MS a place to tell other people with MS what we like about a particular neurologist, what we didn't, what his or her approach to treatment is, and what to expect from an office visit. It is like having a whole family of people with MS scattered across the globe who have "test driven" neurologists specializing in MS and have come back to let you know about their experiences. The thing that really appeals to me is that it is us, people with MS, talking to each other with no interference. There are no ads, no sponsors, and very few rules (actually, only one: you must post the doctor's name). The site administrator (Andrea) even states: "I do not edit reviews! I do not heavily moderate this forum."

Try putting a prospective doc's name in PubMed. PubMed is the National Library of Medicine's database of medical research. Every article in almost every scientific medical journal is listed here. You can search a doctor's name by going to the site (www.pubmed.gov) and typing in the last name and the first initial (no commas) and the words "multiple sclerosis" into the search box. This will tell you about the MS-related research studies the doctor has been involved with.

Don't forget to call your insurance company. Once you have narrowed down the possibilities, you'll want to call your insurance company to make sure it will cover your office visits and treatments. Make sure that your provider is "in network" to help save yourself money from extra charges.

Finally, interview a couple of doctors. Your first appointment with a new doctor is a time to interview and evaluate the doctor on the points that are important to you. Do not hesitate to ask as many questions as you want. Do not feel uncomfortable—after all, these are people who will eventually ask us about our sexual dysfunction, incontinence, and constipation—a couple of questions from us about appointment frequency and best ways to contact him in case of a weekend relapse should not rattle anyone too much. Make sure you get your questions answered: Is there a nurse on call? How often does he want to see you? Will he make a custom treatment plan for you? Can he help coordinate your treatment with other specialists? What does he think about alternative and complementary approaches? Write your questions down before your appointment and assert yourself to make sure they all get answered.

The Real World

Docs love to treat MS. It is a fascinating disease. For this reason, you have something of value to offer the doctor: the experience of treating someone with MS. The doctor must "sell" you her services, approach, and experience. If you are not convinced, take your "fascinating" disease somewhere else.

Have a Productive Conversation with Your Doctor

Doctors have a way of unsettling people. Lawyers, CEOs, and senators lose their bravado and self-confidence when it comes to talking with doctors. Psychologically, we are vulnerable when we are discussing our own health. Intellectually, we don't have the same mastery of the terminology that the doctor has. Physically, we may be sitting in a paper robe with (or without) ties in the back. All of these factors can result in us feeling flustered and nervous during conversations with our doctors—times when we really need to be communicating well and remembering details.

Take Charge

Prepare for your doctor's visit as if it were a job interview or a major presentation. Think about it ahead of time, visualize the visit and set goals.

By preparing for your doctors' visits and making a few attitude shifts, you'll get a lot more out of your medical care. You won't leave confused or with unanswered questions, and you will establish a true partnership with your doctor. Good communication and rapport with your doctor is a key component in your medical care. Having a good relationship with the right doctor can speed diagnosis and treatment as well as reduce a tremendous amount of the stress that surrounds MS.

Be an active patient. Studies have shown that active patients—patients who ask questions—like their doctors better. The studies also show that doctors like these patients better. At first you might think that the doctors would find these patients to be annoying—think about it a little more. Imagine you are a doctor, facing exam room after exam room of patients every day. Each room contains a passive patient who just answers your questions and is intimidated by you. Now, put a patient in one room who is determined to feel better, who asks intelligent questions, and with whom you can share some of your knowledge. That visit is much more exciting and rewarding. You can be that exceptional patient by being curious about your health and MS. Remember, doctors became doctors because they find health and MS fascinating. Share that fascination, ask some questions and be an active patient.

Tell your doctor what kind of patient you are. When I found out that I was carrying twins, I told my obstetrician, "Let me tell you who I am in this pregnancy. I want you to do everything in your power to make this go well. I don't care how much it hurts. I don't care how much it costs. I don't care if statistically it seems unnecessary. I don't care if it only helps in .02% of cases. Do whatever you can to make this pregnancy a success." Boy, did he ever do it all. Without going into gruesome detail, I can tell you that I was monitored, tested, and subjected to every precaution possible, much of it being paid out of pocket and most of it unpleasant. The pregnancy was not fun, but the outcome of healthy twins was worth it. Now, I am a different kind of patient—the kind that tries to negotiate her way out of pap smears and mammograms (to no avail).

The Real World

You have only one primary MS doc, but that doctor has hundreds of patients. Be unique, be memorable. Be that patient that your doctor thinks about after you leave and does a little bit of "extra research" to help.

The point is, doctors often treat people based on their experience with other patients. Every doctor has hundreds or even thousands of patients he sees, and unless you tell him otherwise, he will assume that you are more or less like his other patients. This is normal—doctors don't automatically know your dreams, plans, tolerance level for pain and inconvenience, or willingness to experiment with different approaches. It helps if you condense your feelings about some of these things into a paragraph (it doesn't have to be as dramatic as my "save the pregnancy" speech) and tell your doctor exactly what kind of patient you are.

Prepare for your appointment. We've talked about your attitude toward your doctor, now it is time to focus on action. Treat your doctor's appointments like important business meetings—prepare for them. You probably would have a list of questions ready before going to see any other professionals (an accountant, a lawyer, a realtor), and it just makes sense to get your thoughts and questions organized before seeing your doctor. Don't think that you are overstepping your boundaries—it is respectful to come prepared to an appointment. Make a pledge to yourself to do this before every doctor's appointment. Here are some suggestions for getting prepared:

> ***Step 1: Update your doctor.*** Write out a few bullet points that summarize how you feel and what is happening. Refer to "How to talk to your doctor about your symptoms" from Chapter 3 to make sure that you include relevant information about how your symptoms are affecting you. Be short and to the point, but don't leave out anything that might be important. Be sure to

include any lifestyle adjustments you are making, including changes in diet, exercise, and supplements. Also, let your doctor know about any alternative providers you are seeing, such as acupuncturists, chiropractors, and massage therapists.

Step 2: ***Decide what you want to improve.*** Make a list of anything about your health that you want to improve. You may be surprised what can happen if you just ask. For example, if you let your doctor know that you are having trouble sleeping, he or she may simply change the time of day you take a medication, which may make a big difference. Mention what you would like to improve and see if your doctor can help.

Step 3: ***List any additional questions.*** You may have heard the adage that "there is no such thing as a stupid question." Although I don't believe that is true in every situation, I believe that there is no question about your health that you should be afraid to ask your doctor. They can range from the insignificant-to-most-people-but-a-big-deal-to-me (e.g., does it mean that my brain atrophy is picking up speed if I couldn't finish the crossword puzzle in the Sunday *New York Times?*) to the improbable, but still of concern (e.g., will laser hair removal treatments cause a relapse?). List them all. Then, most importantly, *ask* them all.

Understand your doctor's role. Make sure that you are satisfied in terms of quality of medical care; however, don't expect too much or the wrong things from your doctor. His or her role in your medical care is just that—the medical side of things. Your doctor is not trained in nutrition, behavior change, stress reduction, or counseling. Your doctor may or may not know details about alternative therapies. Expect your doctor to know everything about interpreting the results of diagnostic tests, the medical aspects of your MS, and your treatment. You can ask about the other things, but your doctor may or may not have the answers for you. You may need to find a few other professionals to help you with the in-depth information that you want.

The Real World

Be fair with your doc. The best doctor is the one who says, "I don't know," and refers you to someone else for a particular symptom when she can't manage it herself. You wouldn't go to a divorce lawyer for your corporate merger and you shouldn't expect your MS doc to be able to handle everything.

Take notes. Don't trust yourself to remember everything the doctor says. Jot down key terms and ask the doctor to spell them if you need to.

Don't forget nurses. You may spend more time with the nurses than with the doctor. You can ask a lot of questions while he or she is taking your vital signs. Nurses often have a little bit more time than the doc and may go into greater detail with you. This is especially true in regards to self-care or personal maintenance tips, such as instructions for giving yourself an injection, or how to stay adherent to your medications.

Bring someone with you. That other person can be your notetaker and can remind you of questions that you have. Most importantly, the other person can help you to understand better and recall more accurately what the doctor has said. Also, having someone else along may help you find the resolve to stick to your list and ask all of your questions.

If you think of something you forgot to ask the doctor during your appointment, call the office and ask to talk to a nurse. The nurse can usually answer your question or find out the answer for you and call you back. Don't think that you are bothering the staff—they are there to help you, but it is your job to be precise and concise to make the phone calls efficient for them.

Don't Be Afraid to Get a Second Opinion

Why People Get Second Opinions

There are many reasons that you might want to get a second opinion on a specific symptom or in the overall management of your MS. You may have started thinking about a second opinion after having thoughts similar to some of these:

"I just *can't* believe it—I don't have *that*." Perhaps your doctor has told you that you no longer have relapsing-remitting MS, but that your MS has progressed and is now reclassified as secondary-progressive MS. Maybe you are experiencing a symptom that your doctor thinks may be related to a more serious condition or has nothing to do with MS.

The Real World

Doctors are people, people who can make honest mistakes. For big decisions, it just makes sense to get a second opinion if things are not 100% clear. Don't let feelings of loyalty or worries about offending a doctor get in the way of confirming a decision.

"There must be better options for treating this." You tried, you really tried to make a go of it with the fatigue medication that your doctor prescribed. However, not only were the side effects terrible, there was no noticeable impact on your fatigue. Your doc says this is the best he can do for you. Maybe someone else has other ideas. Or maybe your doctor says that next time you have a relapse, you will have to be hospitalized for the duration of your steroid treatment. You know someone else with MS, however, whose neuro sends a nurse to her house to administer the Solu-Medrol. It might be a good idea to talk to that doctor to see how this service works and if there are certain circumstances where it is not a good idea.

Take Charge

Your health is *yours*. Make your medical care *yours*, too.

"I would like to get the opinion of someone with more experience with my situation." Maybe you just got diagnosed with primary-progressive MS. You really like your neurologist, but he tells you that he has very few patients with PPMS, although he is comfortable having you as a patient. You may want to go talk to someone who specializes in PPMS to confirm some of your questions, even if you return to your neuro. Or, you have been feeling a little depressed lately. Your neurologist has helped you with a bout of depression in the past by giving you medication, but this time you would like to be evaluated by a psychiatrist (preferably one that has experience with MS patients), to see about newer drugs and possibly introducing some psychotherapy into the treatment plan. If you like this new doctor, it is possible that the "second opinion" will turn into a "referral," meaning that the new doctor will take over this part of your care.

Feel Confident in Your Decision to Seek a Second Opinion

There are many people out there who feel like they are cheating on their doctor when they seek a second opinion. I know it can be an awkward situation, unless your doctor brings it up himself. Most doctors, however, will be happy for you to seek a second opinion, as it will probably make you more comfortable with your final decision and even more adherent to the treatment prescribed.

I am not promising that your doctor will have a positive reaction. Occasionally, docs get angry, feeling like the patient doesn't trust their judgment or is searching for something specific that the current doctor doesn't agree with. I even had one person write to me and say that her doctor "fired" her as a patient when she asked for a second opinion.

Script for Asking Your Doc About a Second Opinion

Okay, I know that I can keep telling you that it is your right to get a second opinion and that you have nothing to be nervous about. Clearly, however, you are the one who has to discuss it with your doctor and I won't be there, giving you a thumbs-up sign and whispering, "You go, girl (or boy)." So, I'm going to give you a little script to adapt and practice before you go.

Try something like this:

> "Hey, doc, I have an idea that would make me feel better about this whole thing. Why don't we get another doctor's input on the situation before moving forward? This is kind of a big deal to me and having another person weigh in would really increase my comfort level with any decisions. [Optional: Is there anyone you would recommend to help us with this specific problem?]"

I don't see how anyone could be too offended by an approach such as this. After all, you are just looking for someone to help out "the team." Going in prepared with something like this may prevent you from blurting out something unfortunate in an emotional moment. Even if you are pretty sure that you are done with your neuro or that his decisions are not the right ones for you, words and phrases like "lame," "idiot," "I'd rather eat glass" are just not productive.

Ways to Optimize Your Second Opinion

Gather all of your own medical records and get them to the other doctor in advance. This includes MRI reports and films, doctor's notes, and other test results.

Make sure you get a report on the second doctor's findings. The new doctor might not communicate with your primary neuro (although they are supposed to). Also, you will want this report for your records as well for use conducting any of your own research on the topic.

Make sure the second doctor is board certified in the appropriate specialization. If you are going to go to the trouble of getting a second opinion, it is wise to go to someone who is up on the "latest and greatest" in their field. If you are seeking advice on an MS-specific problem, find someone board certified in neurology. If, however, you are looking for answers to problems around certain symptoms, find someone certified in that field. For instance, for help with urinary incontinence, you would seek certification in urology.

Make sure your insurance will pay. In some cases, especially when surgery or less common treatments are going to be tried, insurance companies will require a second opinion to verify the benefit to the patient and that it is indicated for the condition before agreeing to pay for the treatment or procedure. In other cases, insurance will not pay for a second opinion. Give your insurance company a call to find out.

What About Online Second Opinions?

The Internet never ceases to amaze me. There is now a way to get a second opinion online. If you are, like I was initially, skeptical about this idea, listen up when I tell you that one example of this is Partners Online Specialty Consultations, a service run by Massachusetts General Hospital, Brigham and Women's Hospital, Dana-Farber and Harvard Medical School. Still laughing? Basically, you register and you and your physician fill out some information regarding your medical history and diagnostic tests that have been run. You pay a fee (about $500), wait a week and *voila!* Your second opinion is ready.

As the Web site states, this allows you to: "Have access to premier medical specialists without ever having to leave your home. An online second opinion is a convenient and empowering way for you and your doctor to make educated decisions about your health."

What If Doctors Disagree?

There will be times when your doctors have different opinions. Make sure that you ask specific questions about why they came to the conclusions they did. What evidence did they have? Why does one think a certain procedure is better than another for you? It may be that one doctor is relying solely on studies published in medical journals or how he always does things, while another doctor is basing his recommendations on what you have told him about yourself and how you have responded to treatments in the past. It is never a bad idea to do a little of your own research on your condition, including seeking out a third opinion, before making a decision. In the end, however, you may have to go with your gut when choosing among treatment options or which diagnosis to believe.

Take Charge

Ultimately, *you* will make the decisions about your health care. Be prepared and know what you are doing.

Tame Your Medical Information

Recently, a friend of mine was diagnosed as having lupus. Because of potential side effects of some medications that she was prescribed, she had to have the same test on her eyes that I had undergone when I was having a bout of optic neuritis several years ago. I really wanted to be able to tell her the name of the test, what it was for, what my results were, and where I had it done. Instead, all I could tell her was that it was "a really gross test where there were chains coming from my eyes that I had done in a place that was far away with a really ugly waiting room." (Note: I tried to look this up on the Internet, so that I could satisfy my own curiosity—and, no doubt yours at this point. All that was coming up were disgusting and disturbing animal experimentation sites, so I stopped.)

Take Charge

Don't expect your doctors to read your full medical chart at every visit or to remember what happened to you a year ago. It is your job to keep track of everything and remind your doctor of the specifics of your situation.

An important part of actively participating in your medical care is having control over the huge amount of information about your situation. Clearly, medical information can get out of control pretty quickly, especially with a chronic and complicated condition such as MS. There is information about doctors, procedures, tests, medications, billing and insurance. By having a system to collect and organize all of your health-related information, you will be able to find what you need, when you need it. Having all this information in one place will really help. When you have a relapse, are feeling sick or are panicking about a sudden new symptom, you are very likely to forget some important details. These details could prevent potentially harmful drug interactions or may be used to speed diagnosis. Taking the time to gather your information now will make you feel more in control of your MS and more ready to deal with any health-related situation that may occur.

It's not really that fun to do this, but you will feel proud when you get this together. I recommend trying to do it in a week, with a big reward waiting at the end.

Step 1: Set aside time. Depending on your health care situation, you may need as much as 30 minutes each night this week. Look at your schedule for this week and set aside some chunks of time to complete the steps listed below.

Step 2: ***Create a medical information binder.*** Get a binder to store your medical information. Make sure it is one that will be comfortable (and fashionable) enough to carry to appointments.

Step 3: ***Decide on your emergency contact people.*** Label your first page "Emergency Contacts." Choose three people as your emergency contact people. They should be local and able to get to a hospital and help you if you need it. Be sure to tell each person that you are listing him or her as an emergency contact. Double-check phone numbers and other information. This is important, you will need this information handy when you go to see new docs or if you are admitted to the hospital, in many cases. While you are at it, enter their phone numbers in your cell phone using the names "ICE1," "ICE2" and "ICE3" ("in case of emergency"), as police and paramedics often look for this.

Step 4: ***Write down your current doctors.*** Label the next page "My Doctors." Make a list of all your current doctors and medical providers, along with their telephone numbers and addresses. Be sure to list your doctors (including your neurologist, your primary care physician, your gynecologist, and any other specialists that you see), your dentist, your eye doctor, and any other service providers such as physical therapists. This is also a good place to list the numbers of your pharmacies, including the mail-order one that provides your disease-modifying therapies or other specialty drugs.

Step 5: ***Write down your current diagnoses.*** Title the next page "Diagnoses/Conditions." In addition to your MS, list any medical conditions that you have been diagnosed with. Include things like high blood pressure and high cholesterol, as well as any allergies or illnesses. Try to recall the date of diagnosis. You can estimate if you have to. Give some indication of your status by using words such as "mild," "under control," or "severe."

Step 6: ***Write down your current medications.*** This one is very important. Label the page "Current Medications" and list all the medications you are currently taking and what they are for. List both the commercial and drug names of the medication. Be sure to include the dosage and the number of times a day you take it. Estimate when you first started taking each drug and if (and when) the dosage was changed.

Step 7: ***Write down anything else you are taking.*** Label this page "Non-Prescription Items." If you are taking any vitamins or other supplements, include the name, dosage and frequency just like you did with your medications. You may also describe what the supplement is for and/or what the main ingredients are. Also include non-prescription drugs, such as cold remedies, pain relievers, laxatives, or stool softeners—anything that you take without a prescription. If you are trying any complementary and alternative medicine approaches, make a note of these, especially things like chelation, bee venom therapy, homeopathic remedies, or anything else that enters your body.

Take Charge

You think more about your health than your doctor does. Keep track of your thoughts, health events, and other medical details.

Step 8: ***Record your medical events.*** Make a separate page for each time you had a serious medical event, such as a surgery, a hospitalization, or a prolonged course of treatment, labeled with a reference to that event (for example, "2004 Relapse with Optic Neuritis" or "2006 Insertion of Baclofen Pump"). On these pages, write down any information related to the event: symptoms, diagnosis, date, treating physician, treatment, outcome, medications, dosage, side effects, tests run, and results. Record as many of the details as you can. Be sure to include any related test results on your form and include a copy of them in your binder if you have them. Have one page titled "MRI Scans," and list dates of any MRI scans that you had and make a list of where the films are located or who has the images. If they are on a CD-ROM, you can include them in a sleeve in your binder.

Step 9: Get a box and label it "Medical Information." Whenever you receive a benefits statement in the mail, billing information, or any other piece of paper about your medical management and care, put it in the box. That way you know where everything is. If you need something, you can sort through the box until you find it. It is not an elegant solution, but it will work because it is convenient to do. This is for information that you should save but probably won't need access to. Be sure that test results are placed in your binder immediately—don't put them into your box.

Step 10: Keep your binder current. Don't forget to update your information whenever anything changes. Keep your emergency contacts, test results, current medications, information about your doctors, as well as any other relevant information, up-to-date.

Tips For Making Your Medical Information Binder Complete and Useful

Ask friends and family to help you recall dates, medications, and procedure names. You may need to talk with your doctor or a nurse to complete the task. Just call the office and ask when a good time would be to call back and get some information from your chart. You can also ask for a copy of your medical records, though a nurse may be able to find the information faster than you—she may also be able to read your doctor's handwriting.

The Bottom Line

Your medical care can only be as good as your relationship with your doctor. A good patient-doctor partnership can open up new possibilities for really honing in on the main health concerns that you have and collaborating with your doctor to tackle them strategically, tweaking things as you go along, until the best solution is discovered. A bad relationship (or even a neutral one), however, may lead to important things being overlooked, misdiagnosed, untreated, or not taken seriously. This results in frustration and, ultimately, unnecessary suffering on your part.

Take Charge

The quality of your medical care is in your hands. Your active participation in choosing a doctor, communicating with the doctor, making decisions, and recording your medical history are all major factors in your MS care. Do these things well.

Of course, identifying the right doctor is important. However, the kind of patient that we are also impacts the quality of care that we receive, regardless of how brilliant the doctor may be. In his book, *How Doctors Think* (which I would highly recommend), Jerome Groopman reveals some astounding things about the thought processes of physicians. The most interesting, from the viewpoint of the patient, is that doctors' thinking is not simply a computer-like process of taking in data and spitting out diagnoses and treatment plans.[2] Nope—as it turns out, doctors are people. And just like other people, doctors are influenced by their emotions, including their feelings about their patients and their interactions with them. This is where we come in. Let's face it, doctors cannot be expected to care more about our health and our symptoms than we do.

To that end, we have to step up and show that we are ready to do the work to hold up our end of the partnership. We have to be interested enough in our care to come prepared to appointments with questions, observations, and goals. We have to be thoughtful enough about our symptoms to put the effort in to really think about them in specific terms and be able to give this information to the doctor. Ideally, we should know our medical histories intimately, or at least have a good system of keeping all this information organized so that we can answer questions and even make connections ourselves when looking at the "big picture" of our health. To get the best care possible, the care that we deserve, we need to be active, interested patients—the very kind of patients that got many doctors excited about going into medicine.

5

Don't Let Treatment just Happen

Unlike the treatment chapters in some other books about MS, this is not a chapter full of "shoulds," "musts" or "have tos" directing all readers to immediately start one of the disease-modifying therapies. There are no chirpy little proclamations in here about the miracles of science and the wonderful progress that has been made against MS.

I'll admit it: I don't love it. I am grateful that this medicine exists for me, considering that the best that could be done for those that went before me (and even now for many of those with progressive MS) was "diagnose and *adios*" with a bit of symptom management thrown in. I am fully aware that I am lucky that there is something to try, and that I am fortunate to be able to afford to be on these meds. I am, however, still snarky about the daily injections and the fact that I feel worse each year, despite the fact that I am paying good money to make permanent lipoatrophy dents in my body.

I also have to say that my experience with symptom management has not been that inspirational. For most MS symptoms, it seems like "treatment" means trading in a yucky symptom for slightly-less-yucky medication side effects and calling yourself fortunate.

However, the clinical side of MS is part of the package and cannot be avoided. No matter what your situation is, decisions around treatment are bridges to be acknowledged and crossed. Even if your neuro has told you that your form of MS does not lend itself to treatment, you still have to wrestle with strategies to keep your spasticity, incontinence, or depression at bay. Even if you just will not—*no matter what*—ever be able to imagine giving yourself an injection—fine. Grapple with your reality, determine your course of action, and put it to bed, knowing that you did not passively let things happen to you; but, rather, you made the decision based on the situation at hand.

Take Charge

Don't be passive. If you are going to let a symptom go untreated or try to treat it yourself, let it be an active decision that you stand behind, not the result of procrastination, fear, or laziness.

Regardless of your situation, there is no doubt that decisions around treatment, both disease-modifying therapies and symptom management approaches, can be emotionally-charged and filled with ambivalence. By learning to take charge of your treatment decisions, you will find the solution that is right for you, resulting in better adherence and confidence in your chosen plan of attack.

Consider All Aspects of Treatment

Although it would be great if one of the disease-modifying therapies had a huge margin of advantages over the other drugs in all aspects, this is not the case. Given that we all have unique priorities, risk/benefit perceptions, levels of tolerance of side effects, and different lifestyles, it is virtually impossible to make global recommendations about disease-modifying therapies. Like everything else with MS seems to be, your decision around which of these drugs to take should take into account a bunch of complicated factors, and not be based on a quick mention of statistics from a brochure or the warm glow from a persuasive "educational" company-sponsored luncheon at a fancy hotel.

Make It Better

Don't neglect your emotions and financial situation when choosing a therapy. Your treatment choice needs to be the best fit for you and your lifestyle, not just what might look like a better option according to a research study.

Treatment Overview

Since the mid-1990s, drugs started to be available to people with MS. Referred to as "disease-modifying therapies," these are medications that are prescribed to slow the progression of the disease and delay disability. At the time of my diagnosis, I was told by more than one person that I picked a great time to have MS because of the availability of these drugs. As strange as it sounds, it now looks like the people who will be diagnosed after me will be even "luckier" with their timing, as scientists and pharmaceutical companies are in a race to release the first oral MS therapies.

Forming the first-line of MS drugs, Copaxone, Rebif, Avonex, and Betaseron are often referred to as the "CRAB" or "ABCR" drugs. Copaxone is a substance called glatiramer acetate, which is a compound made up of the same amino acids as those found in myelin. Copaxone is thought to help switch the immune system from causing inflammation around lesions to reducing inflammation, almost by acting as a decoy for harmful T-cells. The other three are made from interferon beta, a protein component that reduces the immune response that can attack nerve cells in your body. All four of these drugs are injected—Copaxone, Betaseron and Rebif subcutaneously and Avonex intramuscularly.

Since 2005, we have had Tysabri (natalizumab), which is a monoclonal antibody that binds to T-cells, making it more difficult for them to move into the brain and spinal cord. Tysabri is linked to a very small number of cases of a very serious viral infection of the brain called progressive multifocal leukoencephalopathy (PML). This caused it to be withdrawn from the market until a rigorous monitoring program could be put in place and is the primary reason that Tysabri is not recommended as a first-line drug. Tysabri is given by monthly infusion.

Novantrone (mitoxantrone) is an antineoplastic, otherwise known as chemotherapeutic agent. Novantrone works in MS by suppressing immune system elements that may attack the myelin. Some neurologists have used other chemotherapy or immunosuppressive drugs for progressive forms of MS, including methotrexate, Imuran (azathioprine), and Cytoxin (cyclophosphamide).

Oral therapies on the horizon include cladribine (Leustatin), which is already in use against leukemias and lymphomas. It has been shown to reduce annualized relapse rates by half, slow disability progression and reduce MRI activity when used for five days twice a year in people with RRMS. The other main oral contender is fingolimod (FTY720). In one study, 70 percent of study participants with RRMS were relapse-free after three years of daily treatment with fingolimod.

Besides these treatments, there are many others in the research pipeline, including novel uses of hormones like estriol and testosterone, biologics (such as intestinal parasites), and a class of MS "vaccines" that alter the immune response in different ways to prevent autoimmune activity.

Finally, in my opinionated opinion, no discussion of MS therapies would be complete without mentioning low-dose naltrexone (LDN). Naltrexone is an opiate agonist which is used to treat narcotic addiction and alcoholism, but has been found by some people to reduce MS progression when used off-label in tiny doses (less than 10% of those used to treat addiction). Although very little formal research has been done on LDN, there is an active group of people with MS (of which I am one) who take LDN and find that many of their symptoms are greatly reduced or even disappear. Others report that their MS progression has completely halted and point to stable MRIs as evidence. Given the dearth of formal studies, however, many neurologists are reluctant to prescribe LDN to their patients.

Type of MS and Severity

There are four types of MS (relapsing-remitting, primary-progressive, secondary-progressive, and progressive-relapsing) and the severity of the disease and level of disability can vary widely within each type. Most of the disease-modifying therapies (Avonex, Rebif, Betaseron, Copaxone, and Tysabri) are for people with relapsing-remitting MS. Tysabri is also used in some situations in progressive types of MS, depending on the doctor. Due to the potential dangers of Tysabri, however, it is only recommended for people who have failed on one or more of the other therapies, and only doctors who participate in the monitoring system (TOUCH) are allowed to prescribe it. In addition, Betaseron is approved for secondary-progressive forms of MS with relapses and Avonex and Copaxone are approved for use in people with a single clinical episode if MRI scans show features consistent with MS. Novantrone is approved only for people with worsening relapsing-remitting MS, secondary-progressive MS, and progressive-relapsing MS. Be sure the treatment that you are considering is a "good fit" for your type of MS.

Your Doctor's Opinion

Your doctor may have a very strong opinion about which therapy he would like to see you on—so strong, in fact, that it leaves little room for discussion. Although I am a big advocate of not being bullied, I also think that there are often very good reasons why a doctor might "insist" on a certain treatment strategy—maybe he had patients that were very similar to you who did very well on a particular drug. He could also have solid grounds for disliking a medication—he may have had a cluster of people experiencing the same "rare" side effect or have been forced to switch too many people off of a drug that they failed to respond to. If your doctor "tells" you what med you "will" be taking, ask him why he feels strongly about it—his reasons may be much more convincing than yours, especially if you were wavering between a couple of treatments and it was coming down to a decision based on a slightly smaller-gauge needle or a tiny statistical difference in annualized relapse rates.

Take Charge

Don't forget to ask your doctor "why?" when he makes a therapy recommendation. His "why" response should be thoughtful and make sense to you.

On the other hand, your doctor may say that it is entirely up to you. In this case, it still doesn't hurt to ask him what he thinks would be the best course for you. I often use the approach of asking, "If I was your sister, what would you recommend and why?" Some docs might not like that question, but it usually elicits an honest opinion.

Necessary Monitoring

Of all of the medications, Copaxone has the fewest requirements for monitoring—basically, people should just watch to make sure that injection sites are healing fine and there is not excessive lipoatrophy (areas where subcutaneous fat is destroyed, leaving permanent "dents" in the skin). Avonex, Rebif, and Betaseron patients are all required to have their liver function monitored at baseline, every month for the first six months of treatment, and at six month intervals thereafter (although I happen to know that some docs do not do this as often as they should, or at all).

Take Charge

Don't expect your doctor's office to call to remind you to schedule your next monitoring appointment. At the end of every visit or treatment, be sure to ask when the next treatment or follow-up visit should be. Don't leave your doc's office or the treatment center without having scheduled that appointment (or at least noting the time frame in your calendar).

The monitoring of Tysabri and Novantrone is the most extensive. Before starting Novantrone, you will need blood tests, an electrocardiogram (EKG), and an echocardiogram. All the tests will be repeated before each treatment. Tysabri can only be given at an infusion center that is registered through the TOUCH program. You will be examined by a doctor or nurse and get an MRI before starting Tysabri, then examined every 3 to 6 months for neurologic changes. You will be asked to review patient safety information and fill out a short survey before each infusion.

Injection Considerations

Each of the CRAB (Copaxone, Rebif, Avonex, and Betaseron) drugs differs in its particular combination of frequency of injections, needle size, and whether the injection is subcutaneous or intramuscular. For many of us, when you come right down to it, the whole injecting thing is a big part of our decision. Some people would choose more frequent injections with a teeny needle over a weekly intramuscular injection and vice versa. Novantrone and Tysabri are both administered intravenously in your doctor's office or in an infusion facility.

Side Effects, Safety, and Lifestyle

This is also a big factor for many people when they are choosing a therapy. Because I was starting therapy as a mother of infant twins, the idea of any downtime due to flu-like symptoms of the interferons was out of the question, so I ended up on Copaxone (the idea of the daily injections of Copaxone was also horrifying, but less so). In my pre-mommy days (back when I cared more about my appearance and had fewer tiny people relying on me), I might have forgone Copaxone because of injection frequency, but also because of possible disfigurement from lipoatrophy (which I now have).

One thing that I do have to say here is it is important to remember that fear and stress count as side effects. I am specifically referring to Tysabri and Novantrone. The deciding factor around these medications for many people may come down to the (1.2 per 10,000) risk of PML (progressive multifocal leukoencephalopathy), the potentially fatal brain disease that has occurred in a small number of people taking Tysabri, or the risk of leukemia (7.4 per 1,000) or cardiac damage with Novantrone. In my opinion, the real bottom line is how you feel about these statistics. Clearly, the odds are in anyone's favor that they will not get these extreme adverse events. However, anxiety and worry are side effects, too. If you think that the risk associated with these drugs will cause a huge amount of stress for you, take that seriously into your equation when deciding whether or not to start on Tysabri or Novantrone.

Do Your Best

After learning everything that you can about your treatment options, make a firm decision and stick with it (until you change your mind).

Effectiveness

This one is not as straightforward as it seems. There are many factors involved with how well you will respond to a particular therapy. For instance, Copaxone seems to take a bit longer to reach full effectiveness (estimates are about 9 months), but studies show that the longer someone is on it, the more effective it is, reaching the same degree of protection as Tysabri (.2 relapses per year or one relapse every five years) after it is taken for 4 years. The high-dose interferon-based drugs may provide quicker protection, but there is the possibility of developing neutralizing antibodies to these drugs, which may reduce the effectiveness. There are also matters of side effects and just fatigue around self-injecting that may reduce personal adherence to a drug, which may influence how well or poorly the drug ultimately does its job.

Know Your Stuff

Neutralizing antibodies (NAbs) are antibodies produced by the body that react with a foreign agent to destroy it or limit its effect. NAbs have been shown to be produced in response to the interferon-based disease-modifying therapies (Avonex, Betaseron, and Rebif) in some people, which can limit their effectiveness.

It's kind of a Catch-22 situation, in that higher doses of interferon (such as Betaseron) are shown to be more effective overall in preventing relapses and slowing disease progression than lower-dose meds (such as Avonex), but higher doses of interferon are also shown in some people to lead to the formation of NAbs, which reduce the effectiveness of the drug. If your interferon-based therapy seems to have stopped working, ask your doctor about testing you for NAbs to determine if switching to non-interferon based therapy might be a smart idea.

Cost

Your treatment decision may be easier if your insurance covers one drug with a copay of 50 dollars per month versus another drug that is not covered and would cost 2,450 dollars each month. At that point, considerations of needle gauge go out the window for most of us. You may also be in a situation where one manufacturer may have a patient assistance program that you qualify for and others don't.

Sticker Shock?

Before MS, I was used to getting a prescription on a piece of paper from my doc and going to my local pharmacy to fill it. Depending on my situation concerning health insurance, I would either pay a $10 or a $25 co-pay. During my nothing-can-happen-to-me days, when I was living carefree without health insurance, I recall shelling out what I thought was the huge amount of 220 dollars for medication that was necessary for my well-being (acne drugs) and thinking, naively, that I was on the far end of the drug cost spectrum.

The world of chronic disease is a big eye-opener when it comes to drug prices, as we need specialty drugs that cost a lot of money. It would be shocking enough to grapple with the idea of paying thousands of dollars for a month's worth of meds, but then we have to get our heads around the fact that this is not just for one month—oh no, those calendar pages keep flipping. In most cases, with the exception of Novantrone, whatever disease-modifying med we end up on is a part of our life for the long-term, that is, until it stops working, we can't tolerate it anymore, or we stop taking it for some other reason. Throw some pricey symptom management treatment in there and we are talking about lots of money for a long time.

The Real World

MS comes with an economic "double-whammy"—you may not be able to work as much as you want *and* you have to find a way to pay for treatment.

It is helpful to have health insurance, but drugs still might be costing quite a bit, due to things like complications with formularies, choice of specialty pharmacies, and weird and unclear "tier classifications," which may mean that we find ourselves paying substantial percentages of drug costs, rather than a fixed co-pay amount. If you have health insurance, the first thing to do is to line up your prescription meds and call your insurance company and see if there is any way to reduce the money that you are paying out of pocket. You might also take a look and see if you are getting generics, which can make a huge difference for some of the symptom management drugs.

DestinationRx (www.destinationrx.com) is a helpful site, which allows you to compare prices on drugs, check out generic options, and manage your list of medications. Just to see what it was all about, I searched Avonex to see what the price differences were and had the following information on prices per month of medication returned: "The least amount your drug costs: $1,978.25. The maximum amount your drug costs: $2,505.68." Interesting information, as this is an annual difference of $6,000 for someone paying out-of-pocket. To see how prices compare at different pharmacies, enter the name of your drug into the search field and click on the correct result in the list that is returned. Then click on the "Pharmacy Pricing" button next to "Options to Consider." A list of pharmacies will be returned, with the prices they charge for a monthly supply of the medication. You can narrow this down by ZIP code for the non-specialty drugs that are available at neighborhood pharmacies.

Prescription drug cards may help ease the pain a little (although the disease-modifying meds are not included). Two to check out are: RxDrugCard (www.rxdrugcard.com) or 888–216–2461, through which members pay a small yearly fee to receive discounts at participating pharmacies; or Together Rx Access Card (www.togetherrxaccess.com) or 800–444–4106, which is free, but limited to people who have no prescription drug coverage and meet certain income guidelines.

Patient assistance programs exist for many of the disease-modifying therapies and other medications. You can check with the manufacturer or you can look at some of the Web sites that have organized much of the information about the various programs in one place in easy-to-search formats, which can help you figure out eligibility and provide application forms for different programs. My favorite ones, for ease of searching and comprehensiveness, are NeedyMeds (www.needymeds.com) and The Partnership for Prescription Assistance (www.pparx.org).

The National Organization for Rare Disorders, or NORD (www.rarediseases.org), also has a very limited number of medication assistance programs for uninsured or underinsured individuals with multiple sclerosis and is worth checking out, mainly for the other interesting information and links about multiple sclerosis and other diseases.

Get a Handle on Your Treatment Options

When it was first suspected that I had MS, the neurologist told his nurse to give me "the literature" on the various disease-modifying therapies. This turned out to be a shopping bag containing four huge packets from drug companies. All of them contained a video and a pretty hefty book. There was also a whole bunch of stuff—post-its, notebooks, lots of highlighters, pens, and a mug.

I watched the videos. They were full of hope and promise. I got sucked in by the happy language, at times thinking, "Why is anyone even worried about finding a cure when these excellent drugs exist?" The videos made injecting oneself look not only possible, but *fun.*

During this time, if you had asked me what I had chosen for my MS disease-modifying therapy, I would have told you the name of the drug featured in the last video I had watched.

Do Your Best

Talk to as many people with MS as you can when making a decision about treatment. Find them at events or online.

Later I went to a "patient education" seminar for one of the drugs. They served a fabulous lunch in a fancy hotel. By this time I was a little more educated about the drugs and I knew that four of the eight people sitting around my round table were not candidates for this therapy, given the type of MS that they had or the questions that they asked. One woman looked up from feeding her husband, and said, "We come to them all. We are hoping that they have something new to say. We don't know what else to do. We know this drug isn't right, but maybe someone in the audience will ask a question that helps us. The doctor just shakes his head when we ask about treatment for my husband."

Figuring out what medical options are available to you can be a challenging task. There may be other drugs that could give you relief from your MS symptoms. Your current disease-modifying therapy might not be the best for you. It may seem that you have exhausted your options, but there just might be something else out there. Many people would say that it is up to your doctor to figure all of this out and that looking at other options is a waste of a patient's time.

Bah, I say. Though there may be things that are clearly wrong for you, there may be things that your doctor hasn't necessarily thought of for your particular case. There may be doctors who are trying different approaches with great success on cases like yours, even if your doctor says there is nothing to be done. It is not about challenging your doctor in a negative or angry way, it is about looking at all of your options. There is a good chance that your doctor will try something new, refer you to someone who is using that therapy on their patients, or at least look into it more if you ask.

It helps to have a system to weed out the false options, to figure out what meds might work well together and make a decision about your approach. I will present some ideas on how to tackle this exploration of what is out there. You will gather some information about the options that are available to you; then you'll do an analysis of each one. By the end of the exercise, you will have a fairly complete list of possibilities, along with your notes and the opinions of some trusted sources. This can be used now or in the future to guide your decision-making process.

First, discuss your options with your doctor. He or she may have very strong opinions about what you should be on. This may be based on past experiences with patients fitting a similar profile as you or may be just a personal preference to start everyone on a certain drug. If your doctor says something along the lines of "We are starting you on Avonex next week," your discussion (and decision-making) may be over. You may also have a type of MS that really limits your treatment options. Nevertheless, I recommend that you still do the research below to see what you are getting into and to make sure that you are comfortable with the treatment plan. Do not hesitate to make another appointment or call your doctor on the phone if you have questions or want to discuss other options. Remember, most things (besides some extreme relapses) in MS are not acute, meaning they do not require you to make a hasty decision. Take your time and make sure you are in agreement with the strategy.

I suspect most doctors fall into the "middle ground" like mine did, setting parameters from within which I could choose. He said that I wasn't really a candidate for Tysabri at this point, and in his opinion, all the CRAB drugs had the same chance of helping me. It was up to me to pick, based on how often I was willing to inject and what side effects I wanted to deal with. (He ignored my preference of "never" and "none.") He has taken the same approach when it comes to symptom management. He will say, "In my opinion . . ." but then listens when I present my side. Usually we end up with a compromise—to try it my way or his way for a little while, agreeing to reassess the situation in the future.

Start by creating your form. On a piece of paper make the following columns: "Medication," "What It Is For" (if it is a disease-modifying therapy or for a specific symptom), "Risks/Side Effects" "Benefits," "Cost," "Miscellaneous." Fill in the columns as you conduct your search.

Look online. I think the first place to start the search is online, if you are comfortable with the Internet. I started my research with looking through the piles of colorful, glossy informational materials provided by the manufacturer (via my physician at the time). Without being too cynical, I have to point out that these companies spend huge amounts of money on marketing. While they are legally bound to not blatantly misrepresent data, the whole job of their expensive print pieces and DVDs is to convince patients to use the featured drugs—not to give you the low down on the treatment. Though it would be refreshing to have someone in one of these videos say, "Listen, I have lumps all over my butt from these hateful injections, and I usually feel like crap for about 24 hours after my shot, but I still think this is the best therapy out there," this will probably not happen soon.

I recommend a two-stage approach to researching these drugs. First, gather the objective facts. Go on MedlinePlus (www.medlineplus.gov) or the National Multiple Sclerosis Society (www.nationalmssociety.org) website to learn the basics of the meds, such as how often to inject them, anticipated side effects, and efficacy. If you want to look deeper into these drugs at this point, go through the exercises in the next section, "Learn more about your meds," to conduct even more in-depth research.

The Real World

There's a lot of crappy nonsense online about MS. Stick to reliable sources until you are confident that you can separate BS from valuable information.

Also, be aware that many drugs prescribed for MS symptoms are used "off-label," so that when you look up your drugs on MedlinePlus.gov or other sites you may find that your symptom is not listed anywhere in the drug's description, which often leads people to wonder if their doc is confused or a mistake has been made. "Off-label" use of drugs means that the medication is prescribed to treat a condition other than the one it was approved for by the Food and Drug Administration (FDA). Clinical trials test drugs against certain symptoms or illnesses, usually in certain age groups, and FDA approval is for these specific problems in this age group. However, once drugs are approved by the FDA, they can be legally prescribed for any reason and to any person. It is up to the doctor to use their professional experience and knowledge when deciding which drugs to use with their various patients. Interestingly, it is illegal to advertise drugs for uses other than those for which they received FDA approval. Many drugs used to manage the symptoms of MS are used off-label, including things like tricyclic antidepressants, such as nortriptyline (Pamelor) and amitriptyline (Elavil) to treat neuropathic pain, or modanifil (Provigil) to lessen MS-related fatigue (labeled as a drug to treat narcolepsy or to help shift workers adjust to their schedules).

For my second (and probably most important) step in my Internet research, I would recommend finding out what "the people" have to say. There are plenty of places to find out about the experiences of people who have tried these drugs. Here are a couple of my favorites:

Revolution health. Found at www.revolutionhealth.com/drugs-treatments, this resource used to be called "RemedyFind." It allows actual people who are using different medications to write in and rate a drug in four areas (perceived effectiveness, tolerability, ease of use, would you recommend?) as well as write in an entry on the drug. Visit it and read what people have to say—it is fascinating. Again, remember that people who have very positive or very negative experiences are more likely to take the time to write to such a site, but the entries still provide pretty interesting perspectives. To get to the relevant part, click on "Drugs and Treatments" in the top menu bar, then enter the name of your drug of interest in the search bar. Click on "Read all [drug name] ratings" under the "user ratings" column when it comes up. Play around on the site—there are ways to limit searches to your specific type of MS or symptom.

Do Your Best

People online can be strange or have completely different ideas than you, but the more opinions you read, the more you will understand. Get stories from more than one place and actively seek out differing points of view.

Askapatient database. You can find this one at www.askapatient.com. Also informative, this site focuses entirely on patient feedback about drugs.

Askapatient.com has a more "homemade" feel than the Revolution Health site, mostly focusing on side effects, although people are asked to submit an overall rating for the drug. An interesting feature of this site is that some people provide e-mail addresses in case you want to ask a question directly.

DailyStrength. Go to www.dailystrength.org. This is also a patient rating site, where people can say if a drug is "working" or "not working." People only post a tiny bit of information on each drug (sample entries for Copaxone include "waste of time" and "I still have site reactions but for the most part no major complaints"). Some really neat features of DailyStrength are that you can send a message to each person, and most people have all of the drugs that they are taking posted under their profiles with comments. The site is a little confusing and requires a little "messing around" on it to get the hang of what is happening. There are, however, pretty interesting discussions going on in the forums.

These sites vary in their activity and thoroughness around specific drugs. For instance, a search on Copaxone gave me the following results: Revolution Health—335 ratings, Askapatient—133 ratings, DailyStrength—965 results; whereas a search on low dose naltrexone (when specifically used for MS) sent back these: Revolution Health—261 ratings, Askapatient—0 ratings, DailyStrength—92 results.

Take Charge

Value the opinions of others, but form your own.

Talk to people. Of course, this is a good thing to do if you have the opportunity. At the time that I was trying to make my decision about disease-modifying therapies, I didn't know anyone else with MS, so surveying several people about their experiences was out of the question. If you are in a support group, however, you can ask for input, opinions, and experiences regarding medications. Prepare yourself for a long session, as people usually love to talk about their medication experiences. Also, keep in mind that some people are very adamant about their choices, so you may be asked about your decision (and find yourself in the position of defending it if your final choice differed from their advice).

Evaluate. Listen, I have been there. I know that we all have different things that we are looking for or trying to avoid when choosing a treatment. If the idea of an intramuscular injection makes you nauseated, scratch Avonex off your list. If your insurance doesn't cover a certain drug, don't bother looking at it any further, unless there are other options for paying for it. There is no point in comparing statistical data on specific drugs if there is an insurmountable barrier to taking some of them. The final choice will be a combination of many factors, including your lifestyle and your doctor agreeing to your treatment plan.

Now, repeat step #1 and talk to your doctor. Tell your doctor your ideas regarding medications. Tell him or her the main reasons for your choices—be specific. However, be prepared to compromise if your doctor has valid reasons for suggesting a different treatment strategy.

A Note About Not Being on Treatment

There are certain illnesses for which refusing treatment is not even a question—for instance, a dangerous bacterial infection that could be cured with a short course of potent antibiotics or an emergency situation where a simple intervention (like a blood transfusion) could save a young life. On the other end of the spectrum are the instances where treatment, although available, is not really a good idea. It might be all but futile and come with an onslaught of terrible quality-of-life-stealing side effects, such as the third attempt at chemotherapy in someone whose cancer has metastasized to various organs and bones.

Multiple sclerosis, as we all know by now, comes with a myriad of I-don't-know and it-depends frustrations around causes, risks, prognosis, symptoms, and disability progression. Without question, this murkiness carries over to the subject of treatment, especially disease-modifying therapies.

In many cases, especially with relapsing-remitting MS, as soon as you are diagnosed with MS (or maybe even before), your neurologist will recommend that you begin therapy with one of the disease-modifying treatments. Your doc, however, will not be able to tell you if these drugs will work in your case. You will face potentially high costs, varying severity of side effects, and the stress and pain of infusions or injections before there is any indication that they are having an effect. Yet, many people, including loved ones, doctors, even other MSers, are surprised and dismayed when some people with MS say "no" or "maybe later" to currently-available disease-modifying therapies.

Take Charge

People you barely know will have an opinion on the treatment vs. no treatment issue. Almost all of them know nothing about MS. Educate the ones that you love and consider their thoughts on the matter. Ignore the rest.

Guess what? It is your choice to go on therapy or not.

The Real World

Beware of future regret if you choose no therapy. If you are the kind of person who looks back, saying "what if?" when something bad happens (like a relapse that resulted in disability), factor that likely future regret into your decision-making process.

Surprised? Listen, I'm glad that we live in an age where this kind of therapy is available to us, but it is still a choice and a commitment. I have chosen to be on therapy, but plenty of people have valid reasons not to be.

However, I will say this: if you decide not to take a disease-modifying therapy, make sure there was thought and volition behind making this choice. The current treatment options may not do well in your risk-benefit analysis and you can say "no" after doing some research and soul-searching. It is far less acceptable, however to just let things happen that interfere with getting on therapy, but leave you wondering "what if?" If your reasons for not being on treatment include things like you can't remember where you left that form, you haven't gotten around to calling that pharmacy back to fill your order, or you don't know if your insurance will cover a particular drug, that is *not* okay. Make a decision that you can own.

The Real World

Make sure that it is you who makes decisions, not your fears, your MS, your friends, or your procrastination. Make your decisions yourself and be proud of them.

Learn More About Your Meds

Last year, when I got my annual physical, my total serum cholesterol was a little high, somewhere in the range of 210. I was offered a statin, Lipitor, but chose to hold off a little, arguing that my impressive (in my mind) HDL to LDL ratio would outweigh the slightly elevated total serum cholesterol. My plan was that I would start exercising and reexamine the situation.

Raise your hand if you are on Lipitor. That is probably a great decision for your cholesterol (and, interestingly, is also being studied to find out if it may help slow MS progression). Now, keep your hands up if you are also taking one of the interferon-based MS drugs (Betaseron, Avonex, or Rebif). Whoops. Anybody with his or her hand still raised, put it down and call your doctors to figure out which one needs to go. As it turns out, Lipitor (and other statins) may block the effect of the interferons. Scientists found this out when they decided that the positive potential impact of statins on MS would probably be a great thing when combined with an interferon, so they combined Lipitor and Rebif.[1] They found that this combo increased disease activity, both that seen on an MRI and clinical symptoms and signs (although a couple of other studies did not support these findings). Now it is recommended that these two drugs not be given at the same time.

There are many examples of possible—even probable—drug interactions that could occur for a person with MS. People with MS often end up taking a cornucopia of meds: From our neurologist we may get disease-modifying drugs and medications for managing symptoms, such as spasticity, fatigue, depression or any of the other MS-related things that plague us. We may have a couple things thrown into the mix to handle non-MS problems, like high cholesterol, blood pressure, or thyroid disorders. I know I don't hesitate to run out and purchase entire drugstore aisles of over-the-counter medications when I have a hint of an allergy or a cold. Then there are the vitamins and supplements that seem innocuous. Many women also take contraceptives to prevent unplanned pregnancies or hormone replacement therapy after menopause. All of these things can interact with each other and with your MS.

Do Your Best

Every medication, even over-the-counter vitamin supplements and remedies, should be carefully tracked for interactions and side effects. Read the labels, search online and ask each and every one of your health providers about your meds.

Given the huge variety of stuff that may be going into our bodies, it is pretty unlikely that any of your doctors are aware of all of the medications or supplements that you are using. Even if they are, it is very difficult for them to keep up with all of the potential interactions that may occur. You cannot rely on the pharmacists' computer alert programs to track it all either, as many of our MS-specific meds are mail-order only and the pharmacist has no way of knowing what types of supplements and over-the-counter stuff we are taking.

Therefore, it is up to you to do some research on the drugs that you are taking or considering taking. I recommend making a little list or chart with the following columns: "Medication/Dosage," "Interactions," "Misc./Special Instructions," "Side Effects," and "Doctor Notes." In the "Medication" column, list the medications you are taking and the dosages. I would include any over-the-counter things you are taking and supplements that are beyond a daily multivitamin (such as St. John's wort or SAM-E).

The "Interactions" column is simple. List those drugs that you are currently taking or considering taking. You can also list things that may come up later, such as certain kinds of antispasticity meds or antidepressants, if these are symptoms that you have that may require medication in the future.

The "Misc./Special Instructions" column holds things that you didn't know about your med, but you discover during your research. These may be instructions that help reduce side effects or increase the effectiveness of the drug, and may include things such as "don't drink grapefruit juice while using this medication" or "take at the same time every day." Also include any contraindications that apply to you specifically, such as: "not recommended for people with high blood pressure" or "should not be used by people with diabetes."

"Side Effects" is where you list those things that you may be experiencing, but didn't know that they were related to any drug until you saw it listed as part of a description of a medication that you are taking. This is also where you make a special note of those potential side effects that are mentioned in conjunction with a warning to "call your doctor immediately if you experience any of these symptoms."

The "Doctor Notes" column is your space to note what you want to mention to your physician and what questions you may have. It is also a place where you can record what his answer was.

Below are the online places that I recommend for starting your research. While it may seem like overkill, I really believe that you should look at more than one place (at the very least MedlinePlus and PDR Health):

MedlinePlus (www.medlineplus.gov): Again, I really love MedlinePlus, which is a service provided by the U.S. government (the National Library of Medicine and the National Institutes of Health). This site tends to include much more detailed information than I have seen anywhere else. You have to read each entry pretty carefully, however, as the authors have lumped information about interactions, contraindications and special instructions together under the heading of "What Special Precautions Should I Follow?" Still, this is the place to start.

PDR Health (www.pdrhealth.com): This is the consumer site maintained by the publishers of *Physician's Desk Reference* (the main drug resource that docs use—it's the big red book that is sitting on their desk or in their Palm Pilot), so it is probably the most up-to-date. This site has nice detailed information about how the drug should be taken, what you should do if you miss a dose, and whether it should be taken with food (also mentioning if food will delay its effects).

Know Your Stuff

When researching treatments (or anything else), look up words you don't know. In Google, just type *define:search term* for a list of definitions.

Drug Interactions Checker: A service on the Drugs.com site (www.drugs.com), this is an incredibly easy way to figure out if all your medications are going to play nicely with each other. All you do is enter the names of all the drugs you are on, including herbals, vitamin and mineral supplements, and over-the-counter medications. Then, click the "Check Interactions" button, and you've got yourself information that would have taken hours to track down any other way. One thing that I *highly recommend* doing is to use the Drug Interactions Checker to see what kind of harm you can do to yourself by combining caffeine, alcohol, and all sorts of illicit drugs (the database lists heroin, methamphetamine, hashish, and cocaine, among others) with each other, as well as with prescription meds and over-the-counter stuff. If you are going to be using these things, *do this research.* It could literally save your life.

Do Your Best

If you dabble in illicit drugs or drink a little—or a lot of—alcohol, that is your business (mostly). However, it is also your business to make sure that these things are not interacting with your medications in a harmful way. Don't be stupid.

Besides finding out which drugs and supplements interact with each other, to what degree they interact, what the mechanism is, and what kinds of problems the interactions might cause, you will also learn which meds are affected by taking them too soon after eating. By registering on the site, you are able to save your medications list so that you can easily change it or check out drugs that you are considering in the future without having to reenter the whole thing. You can also print out the results of your research to show to your doctor. Yep, it is clear that a smart group of people were using their heads (and testing how real people would use the Drug Interaction function) when they put this site together. The rest of the site is also pretty spectacular, as well.

Manufacturer's site: I also like going to the manufacturer's Web site for the prescribing information available to physicians. Usually typing the drug name into your search engine, such as Google or Yahoo, will get you to the site right away—most brand-name medications have their very own site. This is where you are most likely to see any serious warnings first. By looking at the "Full Prescribing Information," you are seeing everything the drug company wants the doctor to know, while avoiding language and images designed to convince you that you need this drug.

If you are *really* interested: Go to PubMed (pubmed.gov will get you there), which is the free online database of medical journal abstracts run by the NIH, and type in your drug's name into the search bar (try it alone and in combination with "multiple sclerosis"). Be prepared to see a large number of pretty obscure studies and scary case reports about the medication.

Now what? First of all, don't overreact to any of the information you have found. Of course, take action right away if you have one of those "contact your doctor immediately" side effects. If you took your Provigil with a glass of grapefruit juice yesterday, however, or you forgot to mention to your doc that you were diagnosed with mitral valve prolapse in the past and it is on the list of contraindications, there is no need to freak out. You do need to ask your doc about it pretty soon, though. Look over your list and compile all the questions that you have. If there are some questions that require an immediate answer, call your doctor's office. Otherwise, you may have to make an appointment to get all of your questions answered.

Monitor Effects (and Side Effects) of Medications

I was really suffering from fatigue—way, *way* beyond the usual for me. It was getting progressively worse and the end was not in sight. So, I asked my doc for some Provigil. I almost skipped out of his office, gleefully clutching the prescription that I was certain was the answer to this problem. I was expecting miracles from the stuff. The first day, I took it and felt so dizzy and nauseated that I had to lay down for about half an hour, after which that feeling passed and—although I couldn't be sure—maybe, *just maybe*, I actually had a little more energy. My midday crash still came, but with less intensity. I went on like this for three days, each day getting a little better.

At the same time, although I was feeling a little less fatigued, I started feeling a little lightheaded toward the end of my days. Also, each morning I was feeling a little "strung out" when I woke up. It was on the fourth day of this when my husband asked me if we had any ham left for a sandwich. Not only did I not know, it was at that moment that I realized I didn't know anything about what was happening in our refrigerator, because I literally had forgotten to eat for *three* days. My husband had not noticed because we were eating in shifts and taking care of our infant twins.

Make It Better

The symptoms of MS and the side effects of MS therapies and symptom management medications all overlap and interact to make a big, complicated mess. Get in control by paying attention to all the factors that make you feel better or worse.

Although the realization that my appetite had completely vanished alarmed me, this revelation did not bring back any desire to eat. In fact, I was disgusted by even the thought of most foods. However, I had enough of an intellectual grasp on physiology to understand that I probably needed to eat something at some point. The only thing I could find that held any appeal was a bag of trail mix, which consisted primarily of peanuts, cashews, raisins, and M&Ms. The perfect food, I thought—a nice mix of carbs and protein, can be eaten with one hand and doesn't require any preparation or cleanup. I stocked up on the stuff. I forced myself to eat a pretty hefty portion of the trail mix whenever I missed a regular meal, which was the vast majority of the time.

Despite a seemingly positive start, my Provigil stopped working for me after those first couple of days. In fact, I started wondering if I felt worse than I had before starting it. I stuck with it, thinking:

(1) it helps other people,

(2) maybe it takes awhile to reach its full effect, and

(3) if this is my fatigue level on this medication, I cannot imagine what it will be if I stop.

It was a miserably hot summer, I was surviving (barely, I felt) on silly trail mix and my stupid medication miracle had failed me. Oh, yeah, and I was taking care of six-month old twins while trying to work from home. Life was crappy, to say the least.

One day, I decided enough was enough. I stopped the Provigil (in a rather sudden, careless way, without consulting my doctor). I didn't feel any worse, because that really wasn't possible. After a week or so, my appetite had not returned, but at least I wasn't completely repulsed by food, so I was able to expand my culinary repertoire beyond the trail mix (which I was, frankly, disgusted by at this point). I started feeling a little more human—still fatigued, mind you—but like maybe I could do this "life" thing. I finally felt good enough to leave the house, so we went to see my aunt so that she could play with the girls and I could lie down if I needed to. I was having a good time, chatting, enjoying my first glass of wine since I had started the Provigil. I grabbed a handful of cocktail peanuts to tide me over until dinner. Within five minutes, I was literally on my knees. All the terrible feelings that had started to recede came back ten-fold. That was the moment that I discovered I had a sensitivity to legumes (the bean family, which also includes peanuts). A little experimentation revealed that beans, soy products (such as tofu) and anything with peanuts brought on MS-like symptoms, accompanied by disorientation, nausea, dizziness, joint pain, headaches, and additional fatigue.

I told this story for a reason. If I had been monitoring how I felt when I started taking the Provigil, I might have: realized that I had lost my appetite much sooner, figured out the connection between consuming the peanuts in the trail mix and feeling so ungodly terrible, been able to stop eating the foods that made me feel so bad, and known whether Provigil worked for me. I'm considering trying another drug for fatigue. This time, you can be sure that I will monitor the effects closely.

Keep a Medication Effects Log

It is extremely important for us to monitor the effects of the medications that we take for our MS symptoms in order to make sure that we are getting the most out of them and that they are the right meds for us. Remember, unlike other disorders, very few problems associated with multiple sclerosis can be measured by quantitative tests that the doctors can run (such as hormone or thyroid levels). Even regular MRIs do not tell the doctor much about the amount of disability we have or symptom-related discomfort that we are experiencing, as these things do not necessarily correlate to the pictures of what is happening in our brains. In the case of most MS symptoms, the doctors rely on our reports of improvement (or no improvement) to decide if or how to continue treatment with these drugs, so it is crucial that we be accurate and provide our doctor with good-quality information.

Take Charge

Do you know all the potential side effects of each of your medications? Maybe something you had been blaming on MS is really a side effect. A simple medication modification from your doctor could lessen some of your symptoms. Discuss any suspected side effects with your doctor.

In addition, side effects of medications can often be lessened by changing simple things, such as the time of day the drugs are taken or splitting doses. It is also possible that what you think might be new MS symptoms are side effects of medication, and vice versa. Logging can help prevent unnecessary suffering.

Using a simple form that you make, you will periodically record when you take your medications, your symptom intensity and duration, as well as note any other factors that may be impacting your symptoms.

Make a list. Write the date at the top of the paper, you'll use at least one sheet per day. Next, draw six columns on the paper—the first four columns should be narrow and the last column wider. The columns should be labeled "Time," "Medication," "Effect," "Symptom," "Severity," and "Other Factors." In the "Time" column, fill in the hours that you are awake, one hour per line (7:00 a.m., 8:00 a.m., and so on). In the "Medication" column, you will write down the medication you take next to the corresponding time. In the "Effect" column, write down anything that you notice that seems related to the medication next to the corresponding time or noting the time. In the "Symptom" column, note the symptoms that you are experiencing. In the "Severity" column, you'll write how severe the symptom is on a scale of 1 to 10 (10 being the worst you could imagine). In the "Other Factors" column, you'll note food you have eaten, activities or exercise that you have engaged in, your stress level, or anything else that might influence the symptom (i.e., "Time: 8:00 a.m.; Medication: Baclofen 20 mg; Effect: 8:25 a.m., slight dizziness and tired feeling; Symptom: spasm in right leg; Severity: 8.5; Other Factors: forgot to eat breakfast before taking meds).

Keep it with you. If you have your Medication Effects Log with you, it will be much easier to make entries. Don't rely on your memory at the end of the day. Jot notes on an index card during the day and enter them on the form each evening if it is easier.

Make entries. Stop at least four times during the day to check in and make entries. The more often you stop and enter observations, the more accurate your Medication Effects Log will be. This is especially important if you are trying to figure out what triggers or helps specific symptoms or side effects. Set a timer or alarm to remind yourself to check in with your symptoms, stress, or energy levels. Try to be as detailed and specific as possible. It will make it easier to see patterns later.

List other factors. Whereas the main columns on your Medication Effects Log are self-explanatory, the "Other Factors" column could be the most important. Here is where you will try to capture and note other things that may influence how you feel. Besides just the medication that you are taking, social situations, food, your mood, and the temperature outside may all impact how you experience a symptom. Be sure to note these things.

Analyze. Analyze your data every couple of days. This will help you to see patterns in the items you are tracking, as well as improve your data input. Look for patterns in the time of day, the duration and severity of symptoms, as well as any potential side effects (or positive effects) from the medications. Take a good look at the other factors and see if you can identify things that make symptoms worse, as well as things that may help.

Make some changes (after discussing with your doctor). While still keeping your Medication Effects Log, make some changes. If you notice that you feel nauseated when you take your medication on an empty stomach, try taking it with food, unless otherwise indicated. If you notice that you lose your appetite after taking the medication, eat your meals before you take it. All these things, however, must be mentioned to your doctor or checked with the nurse to ensure that (1) the effects that you are noticing are not an indication of a serious adverse reaction, and (2) that it is okay to take the meds with or without food, etc. If the medication makes you dizzy for an hour, make sure that you strategically time your morning showers, driving a car, or anything else that could put you (or others) in danger.

To go more in-depth with your Medication Effects Log, try logging everything for a week. In addition to any symptoms you might have, log moods, sleep, energy level, stress level and productivity. By logging everything you can really start to see connections between your behaviors and how you feel. This could give you new ideas about how to improve your health.

Don't forget to log contact with people. Some people can literally cause you pain and stress, while others may lift your mood and help you forget about your symptoms.

With pain or other chronic symptoms, note if there are times during the day when you are not as bothered by them—what is happening during those times? You can use your log to identify both negative and positive factors.

Help Your Meds Help You

Okay, so you have the drugs in your hands (or in your fridge), but just can't get around to getting the medicine into your body. Not only does this (greatly) lower the possibility that the drugs can help you, this lack of adherence also causes all sorts of guilt and stress that is unnecessary. Remember, in this book we are focusing on taking control of our situations, so if you have decided to be on disease-modifying therapy or a medication to help a particular symptom, let's get this fixed. Below are some "barriers to adherence" and ideas to overcome them. Often, just recognizing them in yourself and acknowledging them has a great effect on helping you get past these problems.

Do Your Best

Medications don't work if you don't take them correctly. Missed doses and not following instructions just create more confusion in trying to find the right treatment strategy for you. Take your medicine and take it correctly.

However, before we get into how to get adherence on track, like everything else, we need to know where we want to be before we start going there. In other words, is your goal to be 100 percent adherent to your medication, taking every dose at the same time and dutifully using your alcohol swabs and rotating injection sites? If so, more power to you. Some people can do this, but others need a more "flexible" approach to adherence to be successful. You may need some help giving yourself injections, you may have medications that need to be taken after a meal, but mealtimes vary in your house or don't happen at all on occasion. You may have a special celebration that you want to feel good for, so delay those meds that cause side effects a day so that you can join in the fun.

This is real life, and your adherence goals should take this into account. By this, I mean do the best you can, and feel good about taking care of your body and managing your symptoms. Keeping a healthy attitude toward your treatment will allow you to troubleshoot problems and achieve better adherence than a "perfection or nothing" approach. Of course, some medications require very specific timing to be effective and to decrease side effects or even avoid potential serious problems. You probably know which ones these are, but checking on MedlinePlus under "What should I do if I forget a dose?" will give you a good indication of how tightly you have to control your dosing.

See if any of the reasons following sound like you:

"I don't like needles. At all." The fact that people have to inject themselves with most of the disease-modifying drugs doesn't get mentioned very often in the ads promoting them, or is brushed off with a mention of a fabulous little autoinject device or thin needles. People tend not to like to cause themselves pain. At the time of this writing, none of the current medications is taken orally, so we have the less-than-pleasant choice of subcutaneous or intramuscular injections for those of us taking the older CRAB drugs (Tysabri and Novantrone are given by intravenous infusions). Employing various mind-over-matter techniques, combined with tears and swearing, I have somehow worked through my feelings about self-injecting and brought myself from a hyperventilating needle-phobic to someone who is just bitter about the whole thing.

The Real World

Don't mess with your meds. Yes, they hurt. Yes, the side effects can be terrible. Commit to taking them anyway, if this is what you have decided to do.

Pro-adherence strategy: There are several things you can do to get yourself to the point that you can inject yourself. Not all of these approaches will work for everyone, and you may be someone that continues to have a hard time with injecting—I cannot promise that you will ever reach a point where you do not dread the needle. Nevertheless, they are worth a try.

- A program developed at University of California San Francisco, which is based on cognitive behavioral therapy, has been made available on the National Multiple Sclerosis Society Web site to help people work through their "reluctance" to self-inject. The workbook for patients is entitled *Learning to Self-Inject: A Cognitive-Behavioral Approach to Overcoming Injection Anxiety,* by David Mohr and Darcy Cox. It is meant to be used in conjunction with professional counseling from a nurse or psychologist (there is a manual for professionals also available on the NMSS Web site), but could also be useful as a stand-alone resource by reading it and working through the exercises. Go to nmss.org and enter "self-inject" in the search field, then look for the link to "Workbook—Learning to Self-Inject (.pdf)."

- As skeptical as I am about the cheerleading nature of patient "motivational" materials from the drug manufacturers, I can say that it really does help to use them to learn about proper injection techniques for your meds. For a long time, I was icing the injection site before sticking the needle in. I then found out (by reading a patient newsletter) that this inhibits the medication from spreading around and can damage the skin, and that heat is preferred. After I started giving myself shots immediately following my morning shower, the whole process got easier.

- There are all sorts of things you can do to get in the mood for an injection, such as: creative visualization, deep breathing exercises, or creating a ritual around injecting (mine has included pre-injection music and post-injection M&M rewards). One of the most effective things I do to talk myself into injecting is to look at the clock and say, "It's 7:58. If I inject *right now*, no matter how bad it is, the whole ordeal will be over by 8:00 at the latest."

- Succeed a couple of times. I know that this one is easier said than done, but I think it is the most important aspect of successful injecting. Once you do it a couple of times, you will have the confidence to know that you can keep doing it (and the evidence that you won't die).

"The side effects from these meds can, well, suck." Despite what the drugs can do for some people and the happy pictures of people on mountains and bicycles on the Web pages, some of these drugs are famous for making you feel worse in the immediate future than you would if you didn't take them.

Pro-adherence strategy: A couple of the medications that I have tried caused such disagreeable side effects that I would bitterly wonder when an unpleasant sensation is a side effect and when it is it a main effect of the drug. In the case of a certain anti-fatigue medication, the gross feelings caused by the drug were actually worse than the fatigue that I was trying to treat (and the medication didn't really help the fatigue), so it was a no-brainer to quit taking that particular drug. Here are some things you can do about side effects:

- Monitor your response to the medication—see the section "Monitor effects (and side effects) of medications" in this chapter. This is extremely important, because you need to know if the medication is helping and the details of the side effects that you are experiencing, so that you can discuss the strategy regarding treatment with your doctor. It is possible that the side effects can be lessened by simple measures, such as titrating your medication (meaning starting with a small dose and gradually building up to the desired dosage) or taking your medication with food or at a different time of day. It is also very possible that switching medications may be the best solution for you.

- Some of the disease-modifying meds are famous for causing injection-site reactions. Different people are more prone to these reactions, but if this is something that is happening to you, you can try using warm compresses before the injection followed by cold compresses; being very diligent about rotating injection sites; massaging the site after injecting (immediately for Avonex, Rebif, and Betaseron and waiting at least 24 hours before massaging Copaxone sites); and injecting medications at room temperature.

- The interferon-based disease-modifying therapies (Avonex, Rebif, and Betaseron) are notorious for causing flu-like symptoms, such as fever, chills, sweating, muscle aches, and fatigue, which last for 24 to 36 hours. This side effect is usually the worst after the first injection and progressively lessens with each injection, so that many people find that these side effects are gone, or at least tolerable, after six months (although many people do not). For some people, these effects can be reduced by starting with a low dose and increasing to a full dose gradually—usually over several weeks. This strategy needs to be worked out with your doctor. Taking ibuprofen or acetaminophen a couple hours before your injection and a couple hours after it may help with some of these side effects. Many people time their injections so they don't interfere with their lives as much (on a Friday night, for instance).

- Wait it out. For many people, the side effects disappear or at least become bearable after a couple of months.

"I keep forgetting to take my medications." Isn't it interesting that most of us do not forget things like massage appointments, that there is chocolate cake for dessert, or that we don't have to work because it is Saturday? However, here I am with something I do (or am supposed to do) daily—inject myself—and, as much as it pains me to admit it, I forget it at least a couple of times each month.

Do Your Best

Spend one week focused on achieving perfect adherence. By the last day, it will be a habit.

Pro-adherence strategy: Research has shown that you are much more likely to be adherent to your treatment if you believe in it and really think that it is working. Maybe it would help to think about how long it has been since you had a relapse or focus on the fact that you are still walking unaided or can still do things that you may have doubted you would be able to do this many years from your diagnosis.

If it is truly a matter of the whole thing slipping your mind, you can put into place a number of little reminders. Of course, there is the always-mentioned sticky note solution, or you can set an alarm to go off on your cell phone. I am a big fan of putting the syringes in a place where I cannot possibly overlook them—stuck in my shoes the night before, on top of my toothbrush, or blocking my access to the coffee cups.

The Bottom Line

We all probably know people who are extremely careful about what they eat—only choosing organic fruits and vegetables, performing advanced math to ensure that their carbohydrate to protein ratio is exactly right, and not eating food that was produced in factories that ever used trans fats—yet many of these people take whatever drug is prescribed by their doctors or that they find in the drugstore aisles, no questions asked. On the other hand are the people who smoke a pack and a half of cigarettes each day and wash down their Big Macs with a six-pack of beer, yet refuse to take medication because they don't like to put "that stuff" into their bodies. Then there are the people who carefully think through their treatment plans, research their options, discuss them with their doctors and end up with a bunch of medications that they then only take sporadically or not at all.

In the interest of not being overly judgmental, I will refrain from judging the people that fall into the above categories (at least in print here). I will say, however, that messing with our body's chemistry by putting drugs into it is a pretty serious deal, to be taken, well, seriously. I will also say that not taking advantage of medications that could help us, based on reasons that we haven't even thought through, is also kind of a shame.

We are the stewards of our bodies. For better or for worse, they are a means to the end—if we want to do or be something, our bodies have to be willing and able. You might feel like your body has betrayed you by "getting" MS—indeed it has—your own immune system has attacked the body that it inhabits. However, don't turn your back on your body. Make treatment decisions. Whether you decide "yes" or "no;" whether you decide "I want to, but I can't afford it at the moment;" whether you decide "these side effects are worse than the symptoms I am trying to treat, so I will keep looking," make a decision—and know why you did.

6

Go Off-Road Responsibly

I have three boxes of funky homeopathic stuff sitting about two feet from me as I write this. In a long and boring story that I will spare you the details of, they came to me from Moscow via Paris, but originated in Italy. Aesthetically, they are really, really appealing—cool-looking little glass vials containing amber-colored liquid that you have to snap open and drink, two per day in a specific order. There are 60 of them altogether. I have had them for about six months now. Every so often I open up the box printed with *"SERIE 1"* just to take a look. They don't expire until May 2012, so I can contemplate them leisurely, without the "have to make a decision" clock ticking too loudly. Will I take them? I don't know. I actually cleared this with my doctor (I really did). However, there is something "Alice in Wonderlandesque" about these little vials of liquid that I don't know if I am ready for. What if they work? What if they don't? What if they don't, but I think they do? I ponder that as I picture myself breaking open the first vial (maybe hopeful, maybe skeptical, maybe desperate), then my head starts to hurt and I put the boxes back on my shelf, where just a corner is visible.

I define "off-road" as anything that your doctor hasn't told you about, including not only complementary and alternative medicine approaches, but clinical trials as well. The potential and promise of some of these "therapies" is huge, but the hope often comes with unknown and risky aspects. Clinical trials have their own lure, as there is pretty solid science behind the proposed mechanisms of action when they get to a Phase II or III stage and the potential benefits can be intriguing. Many of these therapies, however, also come with possible hazards, and pretty significant side effects can emerge during the trial phase.

Know Your Stuff

A CAM therapy is basically anything you do for your health that a doctor didn't prescribe or tell you to do. This includes nutrition, vitamins, and prayer, as well as whole systems like acupuncture, massage, and yoga.

This chapter will guide you in researching the modalities that you might be considering, analyze the approach in terms of appropriateness for you, and guide you in discussing these methods with your doctor (even providing a script for the conversation).

So, What the Heck Is CAM, *Really?*

You may be one of those people who thinks that complementary and alternative medicine (CAM) is for hippies, crazies, or crazy hippies. When you think "alternative medicine" you may picture a person (a hippie, usually) with acupuncture needles sticking out of his or her face, alternating taking fistfuls of herbs with long drags from a marijuana cigarette.

Do you ever pray? Do you have a dog? Do you listen to music? Do you ever exercise? Then, you, my friend, are practicing what some people would claim to be CAM.

Make It Better

Health is pretty complicated. There is a lot out there that your doctor doesn't know about. Be safe, but be bold in exploring ways to feel better. Even a few minutes of relief can be worth it on a bad day.

I don't know about your experience, but I was surprised that upon my MS diagnosis, many, many people felt that they were put on this earth to lead me to the cure (almost as many people as needed to tell me about their friend's great aunt who was bedridden with MS until she died a premature death). I am certain that you have noticed that advertisements and promises are everywhere for non-medical "cures." People you barely know are compelled to tell you about a news story of a person who was confined to a wheelchair until they discovered blue-green algae and started wearing magnets in their shoes. Now, according to these wide-eyed and fervent individuals, this formerly-paralyzed person runs Habitat for Humanity in a small African town, when they are not helicopter skiing in the Andes. Even worse than the advice is the judgment that comes when you choose not to pursue the recommended therapy—clearly (in the head of the person offering this valuable information) you are not serious about your health.

The Real World

Avoid any CAM approach that involves going against your doctor's advice or that claims to directly treat or "cure" your MS.

Then you have your doctor, who doesn't understand why you would ever want to try CAM. After all, he is offering you medicines that are *proven* to reduce symptoms or relapses or lesions. Okay, so they work in some people, not all—often with pretty terrible side effects—and cost a lot of money. "So? What's wrong with that?" your puzzled neuro might ask. Many neurologists are thrilled with the advances that they have seen in very recent years, and are often reluctant to see patients spend money and effort on therapies that are scientifically unproven and may even be harmful.

Learn What CAM Is—and Isn't

Complementary and alternative medicine (CAM) covers a variety of therapeutic or preventive health care practices that do not follow generally-accepted medical methods, may not have a scientific explanation for their effectiveness, and are not part of conventional Western medicine.

"Complementary" medical approaches are undertaken *in conjunction* with Western medical treatment (e.g., acupuncture to relieve nausea from chemotherapy-based treatments), whereas "alternative" approaches are used *instead of* other treatments (e.g., biofeedback to relieve spasticity rather than taking medication).

The National Institutes of Health has classified the different types of CAM as follows:

Whole medical systems. These are complete systems of approaching health and addressing health problem. These each have their own histories, theories, and practices, and include such dissimilar approaches as homeopathy, naturopathy, traditional Chinese medicine, and Ayurveda.

Mind-body medicine. The idea behind mind-body approaches is that of harnessing the power of the human mind to affect the function of the body, including to relieve symptoms. This includes many things that are now widely-practiced (many of which are recommended by doctors), such as support groups, cognitive-behavioral therapy, biofeedback, meditation, prayer, and art or music therapy.

Biologically-based practices. This pretty much covers things from nature that you put in your body, such as herbs, foods, and vitamin supplements. Bee venom therapy also falls into this category, as does (at this point in time, in some states) the use of marijuana. I would argue that this category includes procedures and processes for taking things out of your body as well, such as the removal of mercury amalgam fillings and "toxins" through various kinds of detoxification programs or chelation therapy. Dietary regimens could also fall under this classification.

Manipulative and body-based practices. These practices are based on touching the body in some way, such as chiropractic manipulation or massage. Some forms of physical therapy fall into this category, as well as things we can do with our own bodies, like yoga, tai chi, and Pilates.

Energy medicine. Energy therapies involve the use of energy fields. Biofield therapies concentrate on the energy fields that are (according to practitioners of this type of CAM) around and inside our bodies, and include qi gong, Reiki, and therapeutic touch. Bioelectromagnetic-based therapies involve the use of different types of magnets and electricity.

Learn Why Many Doctors Don't Take CAM Seriously

Have you been mocked by a doctor for suggesting that you try a CAM approach? I have. I didn't take it personally. As previously mentioned, many docs have a problem with these methods, as they will often say, because there is usually no scientific evidence that they work. You need to keep in mind that for our peer-reviewed-journal-reading physician friends, "scientific evidence" is gained through multimillion dollar randomized clinical trials. All of the disease-modifying therapies were "proven" effective through this process, as the group of trial partici-pants who took the medications had fewer relapses and less disability than the group of participants taking the placebo. Although most of the drugs used for MS symptom management are prescribed for "off-label" use (meaning that they were not specifically approved for use in MS-specific symptoms), they were still subjected to the necessary rigorous testing needed to gain FDA approval, and usually their use in people with MS is supported by several scientific studies.

Make It Better

If the CAM therapy is harmless, not overly expensive and defi-nitely makes you feel better, then don't worry too much about lack of formal research or data. Anything that makes life better is a good thing, in my opinion.

CAM is different because:

- There is usually not a specific "product" being tested, rather most approaches are based on something a therapist does. Therefore, it is hard to raise enough money to conduct a large-scale trial, as the profits from the success of the therapy would be diffuse, rather than concentrated in one company.

- It is hard to standardize most CAM approaches so that they could even be compared across sites or practitioners.

- Although there are many small studies and case reports of success of some of the individual approaches, it is hard to claim true success, because the studies are too small to ana-lyze for statistical significance, there are no true comparison groups, the endpoints are primarily self-reported data on symptoms (rather than lesions on MRI scans or other bio-markers), the effects from the therapy are usually mild and transient, and the studies are often not rigorous enough to stand up to the scrutiny of the scientific community.

Does That Mean CAM Doesn't Work in MS?

Not necessarily. Admittedly, it is impossible to say that there are CAM approaches that truly slow the progression of MS in large numbers of people, as these claims are mostly based on anecdotal evidence. Even the few larger, long-term studies of dietary approaches, such as the Swank diet, cannot be accepted as "proof" by the mainstream medical community due to virtually unavoidable problems with the design of such a study, such as lack of "blinding," lack of randomization, and huge attrition rates (meaning most people dropped out or died).

Know Your Stuff

The Swank diet is a low-fat diet that some claim can help MS.

However, life with MS is about more than lesions and data and CAM may offer the following benefits:

Symptom relief. Several CAM therapies have shown success in relieving symptoms such as pain, spasticity, or sensory disturbances.

Body awareness. Many of the CAM modalities bring positive attention to your body (and most of them feel good), which may result in a greater appreciation of the things that your body can do, rather than a constant awareness of MS symptoms and how they are making your body malfunction or feel wrong.

Relaxation. In my opinion, this is one of the biggest benefits of many of the approaches—when you relax deeply, your mind quiets, beneficial chemicals (like nitric oxide) are released, while those that can be harmful if circulating for long periods or if levels fluctuate frequently (like cortisol and adrenaline) are reduced, and everything gets a little better.

Know Your Stuff

Proof, in medical research, often depends on studies being blinded (meaning that no one, including the doctors, know who is receiving the treatment) and randomized (people are randomly assigned to the treatment or control groups).

People with MS Use CAM

If you are curious about CAM and thinking about trying it for some relief from your MS symptoms, you are not alone. According to various studies on frequency of CAM use, it appears that at least half of MSers have tried CAM at some point, up to 88% in some parts of the United States. In several studies, most people who reported trying CAM tried more than one modality. The vast majority seem to use CAM as a complement to conventional therapies, with only 10% using it as an alternative to conventional treatment (although, given the number of alternative "cure" books and Web sites about MS, it appears that the majority of people falling into this group are compelled to share their experiences and enthusiasm with the world).

Do Your Best

Do your homework on your CAM therapy before talking to your doctor about it. Know enough details so your doctor can make an informed opinion about whether a CAM therapy is dangerous or not. Bring the labels for supplements, descriptions of therapies, and detailed dietary plans to your next doctor visit. Chances are, if you can present the CAM therapy well, your doctor will see more value in it.

Interestingly, we seem to be pretty naughty as a group about reporting CAM use to our neurologists—surveys show that docs estimate that about 15% of their patients are using CAM—a *slight* difference from the almost 90% who are actually giving it a try.[1]

Reasons People With MS Use (or Don't Use) CAM

Several studies have been conducted to investigate the reasons that people with MS seek out CAM. Many people, understandably, were searching for a "cure," which conventional medicine has still not offered. Some people were trying CAM on the recommendations of their doctor or a friend. Of course, anecdotal evidence or stories in the media got many people interested in different modalities. People often go in search of CAM when their condition starts to worsen—symptoms get more severe, drugs work less well, people feel their control on the situation slipping and want to try something else. The "holistic" or "natural" aspect of CAM also appeals to many people, especially those who are convinced that their MS was caused or worsened by man-made products.

Most Popular CAM Approaches for MS

Because there are no prescriptions written for CAM, we don't seem to mention it to our docs and researchers have not standardized their approach to exploring CAM usage statistics. Therefore, it is hard to give reliable numbers as to percentages of MSers trying different modalities and their reasons for doing so. However, we do know some things that MSers are trying—the approaches used most frequently include nutrition counseling, supplements, herbal therapy, massage, homeopathy, chiropractic care, marijuana usage, meditation, and yoga. There are countless other CAM modalities used by limited numbers of people with MS, such as faith healing, bee sting therapy, and chelation.

The reported reasons for trying different CAM approaches primarily focused on relieving symptoms, including fatigue, pain, numbness, constipation, bladder dysfunction, spasticity, and depression. Between 12 and 50 percent reported that they were trying to slow down MS progression or prevent relapses.

Yoga for MS: CAM That No One Can Argue With

Okay, maybe you're interested in what CAM can do for you, but are not really interested in acupuncture at this time, and modalities like bee venom therapy and hyperbaric oxygen treatments still seem a little out there. Good news—there *is* a CAM approach that you can try on your own, costs very little money and is virtually free of potential side effects. To add to the appeal, yoga has shown benefits against fatigue in people with multiple sclerosis in a fairly rigorous scientific study, unlike most of the other things in the CAM world. Numerous other studies support the use of yoga for non-MS things like easing the symptoms of menopause, dealing with addictions, reducing anxiety and stress, improving respiratory dysfunction in people with chronic obstructive pulmonary disease, and coping with irritable bowel syndrome. Yoga has also been shown to increase balance, improve gait, increase flexibility, and strengthen muscles—things that many of us wouldn't mind tweaking a little.

When I have been dedicated to my yoga practice (which, admittedly, has been sporadic), I have seen amazing differences in my flexibility and strength from week to week. I notice that I hold my body more erect, rather than slumping over my keyboard or leaning on every horizontal surface that I can find. I also sleep better. I'll offer this advice to people just starting out or rediscovering yoga: Stick with it for at least two weeks. I'll be honest: the first couple of sessions won't be pretty—at all. However, before you know it, you'll be doing things that you thought were impossible and feeling pretty darn good about it. Of course, if you have vertigo, severe balance problems, or other things that might make some of the poses a little precarious, talk to your doc before jumping into yoga.

I recommend the book by Loren Martin Fishman and Eric Small, *Yoga and Multiple Sclerosis: A Journey to Health and Healing.* Eric became a serious student of yoga after his MS diagnosis at age 22 in the 1960s. His website (www.yogams.com) contains articles discussing his approach to MS management using yoga, as well as a video that you can purchase for home practice. The exercises in the book and video are accessible to anyone, whether you are in a wheelchair or are one of those people that hangs out in a headstand for relaxation.[2]

If available in your area for your level of ability, I recommend that beginners take a yoga class for a month or two to learn the proper technique, as it can be hard to understand the logistics of the poses until you have seen them in person. An instructor can help make small adjustments in your poses or suggestions that can make a huge difference. After that, you can continue with the class or begin a home practice using a video or audio recording. If you are lucky enough to live in the Los Angeles area, Eric himself teaches adaptive yoga classes where all the students have MS. Just imagine how cool *that* would be.

Explore Your CAM Options

Figuring out what CAM options may be appropriate for your situation and are available to you can be a challenging task. There may be a large number of things that could give you relief from your MS symptoms or help in other areas of your health.

Do Your Best

If you choose CAM, take the time to do a symptom log so you know whether the CAM is working. Don't just dive in without a way of evaluating if the CAM is helping.

Although I'm not going to give specific advice on which complementary and alternative approaches to try for your multiple sclerosis symptoms, the following guidelines and considerations apply to any approach you consider. This goes for those approaches administered by therapists, such as acupuncture, chiropractic or massage therapies, as well as things you might do at home, such as taking supplements. Common sense dictates that some approaches require more rigorous research, especially those that are invasive or potentially dangerous, such as bee venom therapy, removal of mercury amalgam fillings, or chelation therapy. However, even seemingly "harmless" therapies may have their risks. For instance, certain massage or bodywork therapies might not be appropriate if you recently had a chemotherapy-based treatment, due to the increased risk of bruising or damaging the skin. People with balance and proprioception problems should approach some of the yoga modalities with caution. Even some innocent-sounding teas may exacerbate certain symptoms, like fatigue or bladder dysfunction.

By the end of the exercise, you will have a fairly complete list of possibilities, along with your notes and the opinions of some trusted sources. This can be used now or in the future to guide your decision-making process.

Steps for Exploring Your CAM Options

Step 1: Create your form. On a piece of paper make the following columns: "Option," "What It Is For," "Risks," "Costs," "Who Supports It," and "Evidence." As you come across options in your search, write in the information for each column. Don't worry if you can't fill out all the columns, just input what you can.

Step 2: Decide what options you'll consider. There are an amazing number of options and treatments on the market. You need to decide what you will consider right now and what is off the table.

There is no sense in researching approaches that you absolutely would not try at this time in your life. Give some thoughts to what options you are open to and let that help guide you. Regard with extreme skepticism and suspicion any therapists or advertisements that claim their approach can "cure" MS. Do not listen to *anyone* who tells you, or even suggests, that you should discontinue or decrease your disease-modifying drugs or other prescription medications, unless it is your neurologist. People that make the most extreme claims about cures are often offering things that could potentially be harmful (and are probably very expensive).

Step 3: *Look in books for options.* Go to the library or bookstore and find as many books as you can on MS. Just stack them up. Skim through the chapters on CAM approaches and write down suggestions.

I highly recommend *Complementary and Alternative Medicine and Multiple Sclerosis (2nd ed.)* by Allen C. Bowling. It is a comprehensive reference guide to both common and unusual CAM approaches used by people with MS, which includes the controversies surrounding each modality.[3] I am impressed with Dr. Bowling's balanced approach to the different therapies, as well as his inclusion and discussion of nonconventional therapies that many physicians would immediately dismiss or never consider, such as "dental amalgam removal" and "low dose naltrexone"—I originally had the impression that these things were only really discussed in the "MS underground."

Know Your Stuff

Chances are that you are not the first person with MS to try a specific CAM approach. Read books and Web sites to learn from the mistakes and successes of others.

In my opinion, the most important and interesting part of the book is the chapter at the very end, entitled "A Five-Step Approach: Integrating Conventional and Unconventional Medicine." In these few pages, Bowling manages to broaden one's thinking about health, mention current medical approaches, and list those CAM approaches worth considering for a variety of symptoms and overall wellbeing.

Step 4: *Look online for options.* Repeat the same process online. Just spend some time searching the Internet for anything people say helps. Don't forget to go to www.medlineplus.gov for the National Institutes of Health's (NIH) take on your situation.

The National Center for Complementary and Alternative Medicine (NCCAM) is part of the NIH. The NCCAM site (nccam.nih.gov) has articles about the various CAM modalities, CAM-specific warnings, various health conditions that CAM is frequently used for, and CAM clinical trials. NCCAM also runs the NCCAM Clearinghouse, which is a service mandated by Congress to provide information on CAM, including publications and searches of Federal databases of scientific and medical literature, in response to specific requests. The Clearinghouse, however, does not provide medical advice, treatment recommendations, or referrals to practitioners. The Clearinghouse can be contacted by phone at 888–644–6226, by e-mail at info@nccam.nih.gov or by live chat on the NNCAM Web site.

NCCAM also gives the following specific information for Internet sources:

"One database called CAM on PubMed (nccam.nih.gov/research/camonpubmed), developed by NCCAM and the National Library of Medicine, gives citations or abstracts (brief summaries) of the results of scientific studies on CAM. In some cases, it provides links to publishers' Web sites where you may be able to view or obtain the full articles. The articles cited in CAM on PubMed are peer-reviewed—that is, other scientists in the same field have reviewed the article, the data, and the conclusions, and judged them to be accurate and important to the field. Another database, International Bibliographic Information on Dietary Supplements (dietary-supplements.info.nih.gov), is useful for searching the scientific literature on dietary supplements."

*Step 5: **Talk to people for options.*** Start with the National Multiple Sclerosis Society. They can refer you to online information, send you materials, and talk you through some of the options. Go to support groups and ask about each option—you may be amazed to learn what people have tried. You can also call and talk with alternative providers and get their opinions and prices. Look online for forums or websites dealing with specific modalities. Just remember, there is a "selection bias" danger specific to these sources of information, meaning that people who are the most enthusiastic are the most likely to write in, and you might not be getting the whole story.

Step 6: Decide what to explore further. Look over your list. Do any of the options seem appealing? Do you need more information to make a decision? Where can you get that information? If you are considering a medical option, do you need to make an appointment to talk with someone? Look over each entry and write your opinion next to it in the left margin. You could use terms like "need more information," "seems promising," "may be risky," and "explore this option more." Determine how much the therapy will cost, how many sessions are recommended, and how much time and effort will be needed on your part (do a little cost-benefit analysis).

Step 7: Talk to your doctor. This is a must for some of the CAM options, especially those that involve putting something into your body. You can't assume that just because an alternative provider says their supplements are safe that they really are. You want to make sure nothing interferes or interacts with any medication or treatment you are on. It is also possible that your doctor has experience (positive or negative) with patients that have tried this approach, which he or she can share with you. Call and ask to talk to a nurse about what you are considering as a first step. I'll say it again—don't discontinue or alter your prescribed medication regimen in any way without your doctor's approval. This cannot be emphasized enough. It is wonderful if you feel better after starting a CAM approach, keep it that way by working with your doctor.

*Step 8: **Find a provider.*** Once you decide to further explore an option, you'll need to find a provider. Your doctor may also be able to recommend an acupuncturist, chiropractor, or other professional who has experience working with MS. Ask people at different organizations, friends, and other people you know who they would recommend. Find at least two or three providers and interview them. Ask about cost, their experience with your symptoms, whether they are willing to work with your doctor, their approach to MS, and any other questions you might have. Visit their facility. Make sure they are licensed.

Take Charge

Make sure any CAM you try is high quality. Use only skilled, licensed practitioners and buy only from companies that have quality control measures in place.

---

*Step 9: **Before you start:*** Ask yourself what your expectations are. Don't expect miracles, but don't assume that nothing will help either. Also, do not get pressured into CAM therapy by anyone, including well-meaning loved ones.

Script for Asking Your Doctor about CAM

Because I am a big fan of asking for what you want, it is only fair that I should give you a little "script" to use when approaching your doctor about a CAM modality that you may have found and want to try. I will use a specific example that entails asking about homeopathy, because I just did that. I must confess, I didn't prepare my "speech," and in the moment I was way less articulate than I wanted to be. I pretty much just said, "Do you think homeopathy is for idiots?" Here's what I wish I would have said:

"Hey, Doc, there is something I want to try and would like to hear what you have to say about it. I have been looking into homeopathy for helping with some of my MS symptoms, and just to feel better overall. I know that as a clinician, you are more comfortable with therapies backed by clinical trials and statistical proof, but do you have any specific objections to me trying homeopathy? Have any of your patients tried it? What else can you tell me about it?" (If you have any research that you have done on the subject, this is a good time to show it to your doctor.)

Despite my rather lame handling of the subject, my doctor gave me the green light, saying, "Who knows? It might help. Anything that makes you feel better and doesn't hurt you is fine with me." He went on to tell me about a documentary that he had seen about a guy with MS who was "healed" in Lourdes. He said, "It was amazing. The scenery was beautiful. The guy got better, too. Of course, no one took MRIs before and after or any of that, but who cares? The guy felt better." He went on to talk about the placebo effect and CAM, but I appreciated the fact that the bottom line for my doctor was that I feel better, whether science (as he knows it) is behind it or not.

Okay, so my doctor is great. What if your doctor doesn't have such an open attitude to CAM? You have a choice. You can:

(1) Listen to him and not do it;

(2) Argue with him and try to convince him, but take his advice in the end;

(3) Tell him that you respectfully disagree and that you plan to do it anyway; or

(4) Agree with him, but do it anyway.

I pretty much endorse all of these equally, except #4. I have heard too many stories of people getting into medical trouble because they were afraid to mention something to their docs, then ended up having some problem. Because they were embarrassed, they continued to hide what they were doing, prolonging the correct diagnosis.

Don't Be Afraid of Clinical Trials

Okay, call me weird, but I just love "window shopping" for clinical trials. The epidemiologist that I was trained to be loves looking at all of the different study designs. My favorite really geeky thing to do is look at the names of the trials in search of pithy acronyms. Many of us have heard of the BENEFIT study, which was short for "Betaseron in Newly Emerging MS For Initial Treatment Trial." We now have the HALT MS study, aka "High-Dose Immunosuppression and Autologous Transplantation for Multiple Sclerosis Study," a phase II stem cell study. My very, very favorite acronym for a study (mostly for making it sound fun and intriguing), though, is "HINT"— Helminth-Induced Immunomodulation Therapy in Relapsing-Remitting Multiple Sclerosis. In case you still haven't gotten the "hint" (sorry) of what this is about, it is a very cool study that involves using intestinal parasites to reduce relapses in people with MS. See there? Wouldn't you prefer to just say you were participating in the HINT study?

Gratitude Moment

Every treatment we have is the combined work of researchers and volunteers. There should be a memorial to all the people who entered clinical trials so we can have the medication we have today. Take a moment to send them a silent collective "thanks."

On an emotional level, the person with MS in me loves seeing all the ways that researchers are trying to fix me and my problems (including the ones that I might develop someday) or, even better, fig-ure out how to prevent some of the things that might pop up. Some-times I really wonder if a particular trial is a good fit for me. I look at what the researchers are trying to do, where the study sites are, what phase trial it is. Then I see if I am eligible for participation. If I meet inclusion criteria, I might write down some information about the trial to think about for later. So far, that has been where my "participation" in MS clinical trials has ended.

That's okay. I have participated in a clinical trial for something else, and I know that it is a big responsibility, can be time consuming, may be unpleasant, and requires commitment. At the moment, I am not ready to take on that kind of obligation. I am pretty sure that I will par-ticipate in a clinical trial when the time is right, the approach is some-thing I want to try, and the rest of the logistics can fit into my life. I want to be absolutely sure that I can see it through to the end before taking up anyone's time, including my own.

Do Your Best

If you choose to participate in a clinical trial, be an excellent participant. Follow the instructions, report side effects, and keep appointments. The quality of the data that researchers have to work with is a direct result of the quality of the participation of the individuals in the trial.

So, how do people find themselves participating in clinical trials?

The Path from "Person" to "Participant"

Sometimes it's a winding path to finding yourself in a clinical trial, other times it can be a very direct route from "civilian" to "Participant #NDT89279."

Scenario 1: It's something your doctor is already doing. Many neurologists treating people with MS, especially at dedicated MS clinics or centers, are investigators in clinical trials. They might mention that they think it is a good idea for you to consider participating in a certain trial, given your specific situation. Remember, you should *never* feel pressure to enroll in a clinical trial or feel like your care will be compromised if you refuse (or accept).

Scenario 2: You have a specific symptom or problem and your doc refers you (or you find a trial yourself). You may have tried several things for a certain symptom and are still not satisfied with the results. You may have progressive MS and your doctor knows of a study that is trying something new for people with your situation. You may just want to see if you can do better than current therapy.

Scenario 3: You have more vague (but still valid) reasons, such as an interest in the clinical trial process or a desire to help advance MS research. There is a lot of exciting stuff going on in the world of MS research these days. You may want to get involved and be a part of scientific advances that deal with this horrible disease. Keep in mind that there are ways to do this that do not involve taking experimental drugs (see "Participate in an observational trial" in this chapter).

Scenario 4: You read about something and think, "This is it."
I'll admit, when researching and writing about MS research, I get all sorts of excited about this experimental treatment or that one on a pretty regular basis. I go down the path of "what if this really works?" and have all sorts of fantasies about feeling amazing, having a clear MRI, and being a pioneer in MS research (as a participant, of course). Then, like much of my other Internet shopping, I start thinking that it might be too expensive, too risky, too far, too tiring . . . until I eventually convince myself that I would probably get the placebo, anyway. I've noticed that I am the most excited about clinical trials when I am doing my worst and feeling terrible, and my enthusiasm wanes when I get a break and feel better. If something came along at just the right time that sounded interesting, or if I had a specific symptom that was torturing me and I had exhausted all known treatments, I would certainly be open to pursuing participation in a clinical trial that seemed appropriate for me.

Scenario 5: You can't afford regular medical care and think that maybe a clinical trial would be a good way to get treatment. You are not alone in this and it might not be a bad idea. Research has shown that the people who participate in clinical trials tend to do somewhat better than people in a similar place with their disease who are not enrolled, *regardless of whether the experimental treatment works.* Some think that this could be due to the high quality of care provided during clinical studies. I also think that something called the "Hawthorne effect" might be at play here—simply put, it has been observed by researchers that people being studied (thus, given extra attention) seem to feel better.

Things You *Must* Understand About Clinical Trials

At any given time, there are hundreds of clinical trials being conducted on new MS treatments. Each of these trials is in a different stage and examines different factors of MS. Even if you are not actively seeking the opportunity to become a clinical trial participant, it is important for all people with MS to have a grasp of these terms, as this is the language of research and scientific progress.

A 60-second discussion of "phases"

Every new drug that will eventually be put into a human being was first tested extensively in test tubes and petri dishes and in all sorts of ways in a laboratory during the "in vitro" testing stage. As sorry as I am to tell those of you who are squeamish about this sort of thing, extensive animal testing is carried out before the first Phase I trial. The main purpose of a Phase I trial is to determine the safety of the medication, as well as all sorts of scientific stuff like metabolic and pharmacologic actions of the drug in humans. A small number of volunteers (usually between 20 and 80 people) are given the new drug and carefully monitored for reactions and side effects. These trials are often conducted on an inpatient basis for close monitoring.

Phase II trials are designed to investigate the effectiveness of the new medication or procedure, as well as to continue watching for side effects or toxicity and narrow down dosages. The number of participants in these trials is larger, usually between 100 and 300 people, divided into two or more "treatment arms," or groups. One arm is given the treatment and the other arm is given a placebo or other medication.

Phase III trials are only undertaken after successful completion of Phase I and II trials. These trials usually involve thousands of participants (1,500 to 3,000), often in multiple locations and for a longer time period. Phase III trials are designed to provide an in-depth look at how effective this new treatment is, often by comparing it to existing treatments. These trials are also used to see if different dosages are more effective, if the drug works better in combination with another drug, or if a drug used for another condition might work against MS or an MS symptom. Of course, potential side effects and long-term effects are still closely monitored. After a drug has passed through a Phase III trial, an application for FDA approval can be made.

A Phase IV trial is sometimes conducted after FDA approval in order to determine effectiveness and long-term benefits of the drug in a much larger number of people. These are interesting, because they reveal what happens in the "real world" when people take the drug under less controlled circumstances, meaning that people might not be as adherent to the treatment regimen and criteria for who gets the drug are more liberal (in many cases).

Understand exclusion/inclusion criteria (or, who gets to play?)

Every trial will have a list of "inclusion factors." These factors are characteristics of a person or their illness that the researchers use to decide who gets to participate. For trials testing potential treatments for multiple sclerosis, the type of MS you have, if you have used a certain treatment, the level of disability (usually measured as an EDSS number) and other factors will be very specifically laid out. For people of childbearing age, especially women, it is usually mandatory that there are no pregnancies planned during the study period—often it is required that people who are not surgically sterilized use one or two forms of effective birth control. These inclusion and exclusion factors are important so that the researchers can compare the participant within the trial to one another to determine the effects of the medication in similar individuals, as well as protect vulnerable people from entering the trial.

Take Charge

People in clinical trials have rights. You have a right to have anything happening to you during the trial explained to you. You have a right to leave the trial at any time. You have a right to receive information about the study results. There should be a phone number for any questions or problems you have on the informed consent form that you signed. Don't lose that number.

Interestingly, you may notice that certain trials of disease-modifying drug candidates will only include people who have had a certain number of relapses in the recent past (i.e. two relapses in the past 12 months, or one clinically-significant relapse in the past six months). The reason for this is simple: if you are testing a drug against a placebo to see if it prevents relapses, you have to show that there are more relapses in the placebo arm than in the treatment arm. If nobody is having any relapses, the comparison is useless. A case in point is that of Tovaxin, a T-cell vaccine against MS. Unfortunately, it seems that the researchers were unlucky in their randomization. To make a long story short, the people who ended up in the placebo group simply did not have as many relapses as were expected. In addition, the people who ended up in the treatment group tended to have more aggressive disease. Despite the fact that Tovaxin brought the annualized relapse rate down to around 0.2 relapses/year (similar to Tysabri), the comparison between the two groups did not allow the researchers to claim statistically significant reduction in relapses (as the placebo group averaged only .37 relapses/year). This unlucky situation led to the company's stock losing over 90% of its value within hours of announcing the study results.

Understand control groups and placebos (or, what exactly might you be getting?)

A control arm or group is a comparison group. To understand how effective a new medication may be, researchers need to compare it to something, often a placebo or an existing medication. The people in the control group will not be given the new medication. Generally no one knows which group they are in until the trial is finished.

A placebo is a substance given to a study participant that has no known treatment value. Placebos will be made as similar to the actual treatment as possible. If the new medication being studied is in the form of an injection, the placebo will be an injection. If the experimental drug is in pill form, the placebo will be, too. When studying surgical interventions, the placebo might even be "sham" surgery, complete with an incision. The idea is that the study participants and the researchers do not know who is getting the real treatment and who is getting a placebo.

If the medication being studied is for a condition where a medication already exists, however, that medication will often be used instead of a placebo in the control group, which is often the case when new approaches to disease-modifying therapies are tested.

Understand blinded vs. open label (or, who, if anyone, will know what you are getting?)

In a double-blinded trial, neither the researchers nor the participants know which drugs are being taken. An open-label study, on the other hand, is a study in which both the researchers and the participants know which drugs are being taken (and at what dose). These types of studies can still be randomized.

Understand informed consent (or, what are you agreeing to?)

People often think "informed consent" is the document that they have to sign in order to get things moving and get enrolled in the clinical trial, much like a contract between themselves and the researchers.

Informed consent is actually the process that takes place, or is supposed to take place, to ensure that participants are fully aware of everything that is going to happen during the trial before they agree to participate. In a perfect clinical trial world, a potential participant would understand the purpose of the trial, the potential risks and benefits of the trial, and the goals of the research. It would also be clear that a study participant can quit the trial at any time (and for any reason) and is free to ask questions about the research. The informed consent document is a signed, legal document and should be read carefully and fully understood.

Take Charge

You are free to ask anything you want in the informed consent process. The purpose of the process is to make sure that you truly understand the risks and benefits of the study. Read the form and ask questions before signing anything.

In my experience, many people approach the informed consent process much like people who go reluctantly to church or an opera performance—whereas it is possible that the meaning of life is about to be revealed, they are focused on how long the whole thing is taking, wondering if a butterfly needle will be used to draw blood, and pondering the options for a snack once they sign the document and leave the clinic. It is pretty important to tune into this process and get any information that you need to feel comfortable with your decision to participate—or not participate—in the trial.

Get Answers to These Questions Before You Sign Up

The questions below are just to get you started thinking about the different aspects of clinical trials and how they might impact your life. Undoubtedly, you will be adding many of your own questions to this list.

What are the basics of the study design?

- How many people will be participating in this trial?
- Will some people be getting placebo or will the control arm be getting a current therapy?

What is the purpose of the study?

- Is this trial to see if an untried medication is safe?

- Is it a trial of a drug that is already on the market for another use, to find out if it is an effective MS therapy?

- Is it comparing one well-known drug to another well-known drug to see which one is better?

- Is it combining two widely-used drugs to see if they might work more effectively together?

- Is it trying out different doses of the same drug to determine the ratio of benefits to side effects at the different doses?

What are the possible risks and benefits from the medication or treatment?

- What are the known side effects of this drug?

- What are the possible long-term risks from this drug?

- What are the possible short-term benefits?

- What are the possible long-term benefits?

What will I have to do if I participate?

- How will the therapy be administered? Where will I get it?

- What kinds of tests will be run during the trial and how often will this happen? Will they hurt?

- Will I have to be in the hospital at any point during the trial?

- Will I be able to stay on my regular medications?

- Who will be in charge of my regular medical care?

- Will my care change during the trial?

- How long will the trial last?

What can I find out?

- Will I be able to find out results of tests that were run on me and get copies of these (like MRI films)?

- Will I be able to find out if I was on treatment or placebo at the end?

- How can I find out the results of the study?

Will I be paid?

- Will I be reimbursed for expenses, including non-medical expenses, such as lodging, meals, and transportation?

- Will I be reimbursed for expenses necessary to hire a caregiver to accompany me, if medically necessary?

Start Here for MS Clinical Trials

While there are many places to find out about clinical trials, you really only need to go to one source: The Clinical Trials Database (found at www.clinicaltrials.gov). It is a service of the U.S. National Institutes of Health (NIH) and contains information on all sorts of studies (clinical and observational), which are conducted on humans—both federally funded and privately supported—for a wide range of diseases and conditions. At the time of this writing, The Clinical Trials Database listed a total of 70,671 trials, conducted in all 50 States and in 164 countries. The Web site gets over 40 million page views per month and 50,000 visitors daily.

The Web site is easy to use and is designed for you to be able to locate a trial for MS or any other disease by: investigator, type of MS, institution, geographic location, drug name, trial status (not yet recruiting, recruiting, closed, completed), and who is sponsoring the trial.

You can browse lists with these headings or you can get very specific in a search. For instance, you can type "multiple sclerosis AND spasticity AND Maryland" to see which trials are in your area that you might be eligible for.

Each listing contains information about participating institutions and investigators and contact information; inclusion and exclusion criteria; details about the study, including duration, monitoring, outcome measures (what they are looking for); and start and end dates for the study.

Know Your Stuff

You need to understand all the terms in a clinical trial description. Look up any unfamiliar term to make sure you are eligible for the trial and that the treatment is something you are interested in.

The Web site also has good articles for learning about clinical trials in general, including: frequently asked questions about clinical trials, definitions of important clinical trials terms, links to press releases about completed or ongoing trials, and links to abstracts of published results of clinical trials in PubMed.

The National Multiple Sclerosis Society has a news page called "Clinical Trials Alert," which is a nicely presented summary of current clinical trials that are recruiting participants (found at www. nationalmssociety.org, by clicking on the "Clinical Trials" link under the "Research" tab). I find it interesting to scan and see what is new. The descriptions of the trials are written in simple language and include (my favorite part) the rationale of why researchers think this is a good idea. The alerts also include trials that have changed inclusion/exclusion criteria. It is important to be aware that this list represents only a teeny, tiny fraction of the research being conducted on multiple sclerosis (for instance, at the time of this writing, it listed 17 studies, whereas the Clinical Trials Database listed 472 studies, 178 of which were currently recruiting). If you find something that looks interesting here, I would suggest that you go straight to www.clinicalTrials.gov to read the nitty-gritty details.

Rights and Responsibilities of Clinical Trial Participants

Rights of clinical trial participants. Once you are enrolled as a participant, you have certain rights—after all, this is your body that you are "lending" to science. First of all, you have the right to receive information about the study. Pretty much all of the specific "rules" of the clinical trials that you might participate in are outlined in the informed consent document, which should be explained until you understand it. Again, before you sign it, you should ask as many questions as you need to in order to feel like you truly understand everything that is going to happen and feel comfortable with your choice to participate (or not participate) in the trial. It also means that participants should receive any necessary information during the study, such as results of tests that require treatment outside the scope of the study. What this does *not* mean is that the participant has any right to information that might compromise the study (or that the study staff doesn't have), such as how the other people in the study are doing, if you are getting drug or placebo, etc.

You always have the right to withdraw from a study without worrying about compromising your care or making someone, such as your physician, angry. You should have information on how to formally leave a clinical trial and how to get back on your previous treatment, if desired. You always have the right to be treated fairly and with respect throughout the entire clinical trial process. In a trial I participated in, I got the feeling that the doc was a little more cavalier—okay, rude and insensitive—with some of the comments that he made because I was not a regular patient and his relationship with me would be limited, and I now wish I would have said something. You also have the right to be informed when a sponsor is considering stopping the trial and to be told what the reasons for stopping are, especially if they involve a potential safety issue.

You have the right to receive post-study information. This includes, of course, the results of the trial and updates about all adverse events that happen to trial participants, even after the trial concludes, that may be related to trial participation. You are also entitled to know which study arm you were in, that is, if you received the experimental drug or the placebo (or current standard medication) and what the dosage level was. You should also be given access to the results of all tests and copies of MRIs or other documentation that was collected during the study, but you may have to request these specifically.

If the treatment was beneficial, you have the right to continue the treatment if you were in the treatment arm and to switch to the treatment at the appropriate dose if you were in a control or placebo arm.

You also have the right to have all expenses associated with the trial (that is, those that were agreed to in the informed consent document) reimbursed in a timely manner.

Know Your Stuff

Clinical trials are strictly regulated by law. You have rights that *must* be respected.

Responsibilities of clinical trial participants. When you enter a clinical trial, certain things are expected of you and the study is designed with the assumption that people are going to be responsible participants. As someone who has been on both sides of a research study, I can tell you that quite a bit of energy is spent on getting the participants to do things that they agreed to (show up for appointments, log symptoms, take their medications regularly) and a lot of data is compromised because people did not take their participation seriously.

Therefore, if you are a clinical trial participant, you have the responsibility to behave conscientiously. This includes getting to appointments on time, taking the study medications as directed, accurately answering any questions that are asked (with that being said, if you ever feel uncomfortable with a question, don't answer it at all—that is better than making up an answer), maintaining symptom logs, basically doing what you said you would do. You should report to study staff if you did not do these things. It is also your responsibility to make sure that you understand what is going on, even if you have to ask many questions over and over. The study staff does have an obligation to give you this information, but they won't know you don't understand it unless you tell them.

If you are going to stop taking your medications for any reason, or if you are adding something new to your treatment regimen (including things prescribed by your regular doctor for related or non-related things) or are planning to have surgery, you must tell the study staff before you do any of these things. They should also be informed of any illness or accident that you have during the trial.

Find Out the Implications of Clinical Trial Participation on Your Health Insurance Coverage

It is important to find out exactly which treatments or procedures will be paid for by your insurance company before you sign up for a clinical trial. As it turns out, some insurance plans will deny payment for treatment received during a clinical trial.

This was a confusing issue to me, as I assumed that all care given to me in a clinical trial was free, meaning paid for by the trial sponsors and not my problem. That is true for the most part—when someone becomes a participant in a clinical trial, the cost of tests, procedures, study drugs, extra doctor visits, and any research directly related to the study itself is covered by the group that sponsors the clinical trial. Often the study will even pay for transportation.

In some states, however, coverage of *basic medical treatment* can be denied to those who enroll in a clinical trial, if the treatment being tested is considered "experimental" or "investigational." Again, in some of these cases, health insurance may not cover some of the costs of what is actually routine care. This "routine care" includes things like doctor visits, procedures and tests that you would have received anyway, even if you were not taking part in a clinical trial.

Many people who participate in clinical trials have health insurance that pays for at least part of their care. A number of states have passed legislation requiring health plans to pay the cost of routine medical care for patients in clinical trials. Both Medicare and the Veterans Administration will pay for treatment received in clinical trials, with some restrictions. To find out what the insurance implications are for you, first talk to the study staff—they will help you weed through some of the specifics about any costs involved in the trial and who is responsible for them. You should also double-check with your insurance company before enrolling, just to make sure that you fully understand their policies on clinical trials and specifically the one that you are planning to participate in.

Consider Participating in a "Beginner" Clinical Trial

If you think you might be interested in a clinical trial, but aren't quite sure that it is right for you, you can get your feet wet by participating in an observational study. This can be a prospective study where there is no intervention assigned, such as medicine, physical therapy, or lifestyle changes, but you are followed for a set amount of time forward to see what happens to you. In a retrospective study, you may be asked a number of questions about things that happened to you or that you did in the past, such as your smoking history, illnesses that you may have had, vaccines you may have gotten, or past eating habits. You could also sign up for a trial that does not involve medication (or surgery), but uses another type of intervention, such as a computer program for cognitive dysfunction or cognitive behavioral therapy for fatigue. Do be aware, however, that some of these trials may involve giving blood or getting an MRI scan (or several).

These kinds of trials give you a chance to contribute to research around multiple sclerosis without much risk to yourself. They also allow you to experience trial participation to see what it is like. Even the very simplest trial usually involves answering a huge number of questions that can get tedious and seem a little intrusive at times. I participated in a study about MS in mothers of young children that involved filling out a long questionnaire and getting my husband to complete one, which kind of dampened my enthusiasm to participate in a more involved trial.

I do recommend that everyone with MS join the NARCOMS (North American Research Committee on Multiple Sclerosis) Registry (www.narcoms.org), a database with an enrollment of over 34,000 people with MS. The NARCOMS Registry is used both to take a look at what is happening with MS in North America, and also to recruit participants for clinical trials. I have registered. It takes about 30 minutes and you will be asked questions about demographic information, MS-related medical history, any treatments you are on (both disease-modifying therapies and symptom management), health care utilization, and a "series of patient-assessed performance scales that reflect disability in eight domains of function." You can complete the survey online or participate by mail, and are expected to fill out quarterly updates. As a bonus, you receive a free subscription to the printed version of *Multiple Sclerosis Quarterly Report*, a high-quality publication that contains articles about different aspects of life with MS, as well as listings of MS-specific clinical trials.

The Bottom Line

It would be great if there was something that worked for everyone with MS, stopping disease progression and making symptoms disappear. There isn't. For some people, the available medications will work wonders and they will find exactly the right combination of drugs by working closely with their neurologists to produce spectacular results. Many of us with MS, however, will get to a point where we have to accept that conventional medicine has taken us as far as it can in solving certain problems. At that point, some people will decide that "this is good enough" and that they are grateful for the improvement that they have seen (or angry that it isn't any better) and stick with the meds that they are on, perhaps keeping an eye on the news for pharmaceutical breakthroughs.

Make It Better

Explore. Do what you can to make yourself better, but be safe. Most importantly, if you do try something, know how you will evaluate the effects. Explore, but make sure you learn (and stay safe) as you do.

Then there are the people that stand at the crossroads and tell themselves that, no, this is just not good enough, and decide that they are ready to step outside of the box and see what else is out there in the world. This may lead them to try a complementary or alternative approach or it may result in these people participating in clinical trials.

Either path—that of informed acceptance of current reality or of questing for something else—is valid, as long as it is done safely and each person is consciously proceeding down the path that he or she has chosen. This implies that we have all done our research, searched our souls, and are committed to doing what we think is right for our bodies.

7

Be Prepared to Enjoy Life

Something happens to me every year with such regularity that even I am surprised that I am surprised—sometime in the middle of November, I start talking about how dark it is. It goes something like, "Wow. It sure seems to be getting dark early. Did you notice how dark it is now? I mean, it used to be light at 6:00 pm, and now it is dark. I know it gets darker earlier this time of year, but man, this is *dark*. Yep, way darker than I remember."

Judging from the fact that I get blindsided by the change of seasons, you might think that I am often caught unprepared for all sorts of things. You would be right in your assumptions that, for me, holidays seem to spring out of nowhere and birthday gifts often consist of an I.O.U. note for something that I simply forgot to buy.

When it comes to the very real and very unpredictable "surprises" that MS can deliver, however, I feel pretty prepared. The bombshells that can be dropped by MS can take the form of a relapse that literally brings you to your knees, or a symptom that has suddenly worsened enough to exceed your current coping strategies and render the effects of medications inadequate. You may have to drop everything to see your doc, get an MRI scan, and sign up for a lovely five-day Solu-Medrol "trip" that you had not been planning on at all. In a less dramatic, but equally debilitating situation, you might not be able to get out of bed due to fatigue. You may have to quickly figure out how to stay mobile if your spasticity or muscle weakness unexpectedly and suddenly worsens enough to make your cane insufficient.

These unexpected MS surprises are extra special, because they are *in addition* to the challenges of the standard symptoms that we deal with constantly. We know that these demons lurk, yet our tightly-choreographed lives can get derailed pretty easily when our MS decides to be dramatic. It's a terrible cycle that can look like this:

(1) you wake up to find out your legs don't want to carry you around today;

(2) you then start panicking about who is going to take over the sales presentation at work and make sure the kids get to school;

(3) you make frantic phone calls to work and your spouse rearranges his/her schedule to take care of the kids;

(4) while you are listening to the litany of "Mommy/Daddy doesn't do it like *that*" coming from the kitchen, you are dialing your doctor to get an appointment;

(5) your spouse further rearranges his/her schedule to take you to the appointment, which turns into eight appointments over the next week (an initial visit to the neuro, a trip to the MRI imaging center, a follow-up appointment with the neuro, and five excursions to the infusion center for daily infusions of Solu-Medrol);

(6) without your full attention, the house degrades and things at work get confused just enough to cause some Solu-Medrol induced "'roid rage" in you . . . . All of this is happening at a time when many "experts" (usually people without MS) say that we really need to relax, because stress makes MS symptoms and relapses worse. As if.

The Real World

"'Roid rage" (aggression) is often a side effect of Solu-Medrol treatment. This is a perfect example of the need to understand and remember the side effects (especially mood-altering ones) of medication. When on steroids, you may experience paranoia, anger, irritation, and extreme anxiety. You need to remind yourself constantly that these are side effects. It helps if your loved ones know about the side effects and can remind you, too.

I tried to emphasize the importance of avoiding loud, annoying, stressful situations to one of my relatives during his course of Solu-Medrol. He decided to test the theory by taking his family to Chuck E. Cheese's. The result wasn't good.

The other component to living a life in a state of readiness is to be able to roll with the non-MS stressors that might come our way. Like everybody else, things happen to us—little things that require us to rearrange our schedules or big things that require us to rearrange our lives. Being able to identify stressors and separate reality from emotions will go a long way in helping us cope with surprises or annoyances in a calm manner, which will also help our MS stay "calm."

There are also events that we plan—trips, pregnancies, moves, substantial life changes. By thinking ahead strategically, we can minimize the interference in these events that might come from our MS, and lessen the impact of these changes on our MS.

Plan for a Relapse or Symptom Worsening

It's true that most people have forgotten how to be sick. Although they should be resting, they try to do their work from home, take care of a family, and maintain a house without slowing down. The experts are right: when you are under stress, your body doesn't heal as well as it could, due to circulating cortisol and other stress hormones, as well as indirect effects of poor sleep quality and other negative impacts of stress. You can mitigate this cycle by putting in some effort before a relapse comes or your symptoms get worse to ensure that the important things get done, even if you need to take it easy for a while. It might seem a little strange to plan out your life like this, but you will also have the peace of mind that comes from knowing that you have a plan. Think of it as a form of insurance.

Take Charge

You know you are going to have bad days and bad weeks. Get started planning for them to lessen stress, both in the future and right now.

To get yourself ready, you'll make lists and create "action items" for all your tasks and obligations. Depending on your situation, your lists may be long or short. For each item, you'll indicate who can do it, how they should proceed, and what they will need. When you finish, you'll have a comprehensive master plan, covering everything from work obligations to taking care of your home. As a bonus, you'll also have a special care package to make your recovery process more pleasant.

Here are some steps to plan for a relapse or symptom worsening:

Step 1: Make a form. Make four columns on a piece of paper. Label them "Tasks/Needs," "Action," "Delegate," and "Preparation." You'll need a separate sheet for each of the lists described below.

Step 2: List all that you do. Prepare to be shocked when you see everyone and everything that depends on you. Write down everything that you do—all your responsibilities, obligations, and tasks, basically identifying everything you need to plan for.

List out-of-the-house obligations. In the "Tasks/Needs" column, list everything that you are responsible for outside of the house. List all your work responsibilities, as well as your committee or volunteer roles. Do you carpool? Do you help out at your church? Do you answer phones at work? Do you run meetings? Imagine that you are suddenly unable to drive or cannot come into work for a week—what needs to be done? Make the list long and detailed. Spend some time visualizing everything you are involved in and responsible for.

List home/family responsibilities. What do you do at home? Do you cook, clean, shop? Are you the one who pays bills? Mows the lawn? Walks the dog? Do you take care of children? Do you take the kids to school every day? Don't underestimate all the things you do at home. Be sure to note even small things so they are not forgotten—a situation that could cause tension in your home as you try to deal with increased symptoms, treatment, and recovery.

List self needs. Imagine that you are on bed rest for a week. What would you need? You'll definitely require food and something to drink. Will you need someone to take you to the doctor? To help you with medications? Will you need someone during the day, or could you manage on your own? What would make it as pleasant as possible for you—DVDs of your favorite movies, books-on-tape, music? Write down all your needs and wants—don't be shy and be specific.

Make It Better

Don't forget to take care of yourself. Every small improvement counts towards your recovery.

Some tips for making your lists useful include:

- Don't write big, general statements such as "take care of the kids" or "run my company." You're going to have to do some work and write out the detailed tasks. The idea later will be to develop solutions for each of those tasks so you won't have to worry about anything.

- Look over your calendar and old to-do lists to jog your memory. Go through a typical week in your mind to identify all your tasks and responsibilities.

- Plan on making one of the three lists during each of the next few days. You'll want to spend about 30 minutes really concentrating and getting all the details down.

- Ask your spouse, coworkers, partner, or good friend to help you with the lists. Sometimes it may be difficult to think of all the people who rely on you and all the things you are responsible for. Ask these folks if you have covered things fully. As a bonus, people may be shocked when they hear all of the things that you do.

Step 3. Eliminate things. Look over your lists. If there are any tasks or items that would automatically get done without you, cross them off. These are things that you would honestly not even think about if you were not there. At home, cleaning the toilets, vacuuming, and dusting can wait indefinitely. However, be sure that you only cross off tasks that won't cause you worry or bother you if they are undone for a while.

Step 4. Identify things that can be handled by phone calls or e-mail. Look over the remaining items. In the column labeled "Action," write the word "call" or "e-mail" next to any item that could be addressed with a simple phone call or e-mail message. For example, you might simply need to call work and they could cover for you in your absence. Maybe you just need to call and tell a friend to take over a committee meeting. Write the name of the person/place to call next to the word "call" and include the phone number. After the word "e-mail," write out the e-mail address (don't rely on the address book of your computer or e-mail account to provide them when they are needed—someone else may have to send these e-mails).

Step 5. ***Delegate.***Next, write the name of the person who needs to do the action in the "Delegate" column. Think about each item carefully—who could you delegate these tasks to? Maybe a good friend or your spouse could call people for you. Maybe you could simply send an e-mail to someone asking them to take some actions for you. Maybe a coworker could help out.

Don't use just one other person for all the items. You may be writing your spouse's or your best friend's name a few too many times. Try not to rely on these people too much—you'll need them for emotional and other types of support, too. Write down several people that could do a task—give yourself options and don't be afraid to rely on other people. People like to be asked to help in a crisis.

Don't be afraid to hire out. Look over the remaining tasks. These are the things that still need to be done. Write the word "hire" next to any task that you can afford to hire someone to do. Can the teenager next door mow the lawn for you? Can you order take-out food for the family each night? Can you find a babysitter to help out in the afternoons? After the word "hire," write the name and phone number of the person or company you would hire.

Step 6. ***Get prepared.*** For the remaining items, fill in the "Action" column by writing a verb next to each item. Some of the items on your list may not be easily handed over to someone else. If any of the items require advance preparation, jot a note of what you need to do in the "Prepare" column. For example, if you are a teacher, you might need to create a generic substitute teacher lesson plan for an emergency. Think about what you do at work—what would help a coworker easily take over your tasks for a while? What about at home—do you need to turn a form in at the school so your mother can pick up the kids? Make all of the tasks "automatic." Print out maps. Print out take-out menus and circle items. Write down a generic grocery list and get some cash that you can give to someone. Think of ways to make it easy for people to help you.

You may have to show someone how to do a particular task. Write the word "train" next to that item in the "Prepare" column. Maybe someone will be put in charge of your accounts and will need training and tips for dealing with specific clients. Can your husband operate the washing machine (don't laugh)? Write out any instructions and place them in a folder.

Be sure to do anything that you wrote in the "Prepare" column as soon as possible and check it off.

Don't feel that giving detailed instructions and delegating is selfish or bossy. You are making the lives of other people easier—they would have to do these things anyway if you were not there, you're just making it efficient for them.

Take Charge

Plan, plan, plan. You can eliminate a huge portion of the stress surrounding a relapse through careful planning.

Step 7. Do some extra planning for "self care."

Think about medical care. Review your self-care list and make sure you have included everything that you will need regarding your medical care. Do you have an easy way to get your medications? Who will pick them up? Who can take you to doctors' appointments? What other items do you need? Make sure they are written down. Next to each, jot down who will help you and how it will get done. Be sure to include phone numbers for pharmacies and doctors, as well as other key pieces of information.

Don't forget that you have to eat. Make sure your list includes foods that you like to eat and drinks that you like. Include brand names and flavors so someone can bring you just the right thing. Also include restaurants that you like and your favorite take-out order.

Throw in a little pampering. Next, mark any things that you have listed that will help you emotionally or keep your mind occupied. Make a self-care package by getting all the items (DVDs, books, music, computer games, an eye pillow, aromatherapy) and put them in one place. Take a day and actually assemble your care package. Have fun thinking about things that you would just love—give yourself a budget and go shopping. Then hide them away and don't use the items. If you are recovering from a relapse or have a symptom flare-up, you'll look forward to opening this box. It can really help.

Step 8. ***Alert the troops.*** Talk to people if you are not sure they will be available to help when you need them. Don't surprise them with requests when you need them. If they agree beforehand there will be no awkwardness. Just explain that you are trying to get everything ready just in case, so you won't worry. By the way, don't forget to thank everyone when you feel better.

Step 9. ***Create a master plan.*** By now you have several pages of lists, items and ideas—you just need to pull it all together. If necessary, recopy or type up your lists so that someone else can read them. Make separate instruction sheets for critical people. Be sure to include everything they need to take action. Put all these sheets together in one place, as well as any additional documents, instructions, menus, or other information that will be helpful.

Test your master plan on a few people—make sure they understand what you are asking someone to do. Your spouse or a good friend can really help you find the right words to explain what you mean. Now, give yourself a little pat on the back or a small reward for putting in the effort to ensure that you have taken a huge amount of stress out of the equation in the case of a relapse or symptom worsening.

Deconstruct Stress

I imagine that most people can relate to having that buzzy, annoying feeling of stress at times when everything is actually just fine, MS-wise—your symptoms are stable and your meds are treating you well. Even though life is normal, little things get turned into looming mountains of worry and any wrong move could cause an avalanche. For instance, in about a month from writing this, my twins are about to embark on their first week of day camp. For some reason, I am a fretting mess over what I will pack in their lunches. Meanwhile, there are very real, much larger things in my life that could be a much more legitimate source of stress, but that I am coping with just fine. The reality is that stress, like other emotions, is not objective, but is a result of very complex subconscious responses to our perceptions of situations. Because of this, to effectively combat stress and reduce the negative physical aspects of stress, one must take a look deeper into the immediate situation or circumstances and identify what is really plucking at the primal parts of our brain—those regions that lay beyond simple reason and logic. You may find that certain things cause surprising visceral reactions as your mind takes you on a voyage that you are largely unaware of, but that results in a feeling of stress.

Know Your Stuff

MS and stress interact through mechanisms like fluctuations in cortisol levels and the resulting impact of this on the immune system. Stress has been shown to make MS symptoms worse and is even linked to triggering relapses in some studies.

Plenty of things contribute to stress, but one of the main things is not feeling in control of your situation, whether it is a tiny moment in your life (you get confused in the grocery aisle) or bigger events, such as trying to decide whether or not to have a baby. Almost any situation can be dealt with in a calm, effective way if you feel like you know what might happen and have some tactics to deal with the possibilities. The first step in learning to approach life strategically is to be able to identify stress triggers accurately, and to separate your stressors (those things that cause you stress) from your reactions to them—only then will you be able to figure out how to combat and minimize your response to these triggers.

Steps for keeping a stress log and deconstructing stress:

Go on a stressor hunt. As you go through your day, try to recognize stressors that you encounter, no matter how small. Perhaps an old dent in your car door causes you a little bit of stress when you see your car each day. Does a coworker's work style really bother you? Are you watching the number of syringes in your refrigerator dwindle, but haven't yet placed the call to arrange your next shipment?

Assess your reactions. When you recognize a stressor, immediately describe your feelings. For example, a stressor might make you feel tired, overwhelmed, panicked, angry, embarrassed, or anxious. Again, make sure that you note these things immediately—emotions can be fleeting or can change quickly into reactions against other things.

Now that you have started to identify stressors and your reactions to them, you need to take a stab at figuring out why you had those reactions. The word "stress" is so vague and overused, it no longer means anything. People talk to each other about how "stressed" they are, but rarely get any deeper than that. This is a real problem, because we usually stop digging for the real roots of our stress, which makes it pretty much impossible to address in a meaningful way.

Here are the steps to deconstruct stress:

Ban the word "stress." Use the word "stress" as little as possible in your thinking. Try to find other words or phrases to describe what you are feeling. Do not simply substitute another label for the word "stress." For example, do not simply switch to the word "overwhelmed" in your speech and thoughts. Take things deeper and figure out what is really bothering you and why that might be.

Don't blame. It can be easy to start blaming others for your stress. Make it about you—after all, you are the one with the stress. Use the word "I" immediately after "because" to keep the focus on yourself.

Use "because." When you are thinking or talking about your stress, use the word "because" to force yourself to attach a reason to your feeling. Use the following formula: "I am feeling [blank] because I [blank]." When I look at my "camp lunch" anxiety using this approach, I would end up with something like: "I am feeling sad and a little scared because I am leaving the girls in a group setting for the first time and I am worried that they won't like it, won't eat, and won't understand why they are there." Now, this gives me something to sink my teeth into and really deal with, rather than continuing to focus on whether Cheese Nips or Goldfish are a better choice.

Make Life Enjoyable

Getting pleasure out of everyday things, especially the things that we have to do, is one of the secrets to happiness. Unfortunately, we spend a lot of time looking forward to events that will happen in the future (and rarely turn out as good as we had pictured them), while slogging through daily life without noticing the details. Taking a week to invest a little effort into "upgrading" our daily tasks can give great returns. Doing this is easy:

Make It Better

The world is filled with wonderful things, try to bring as many of them into your life as you can. Think about smells, sights, and sounds that can make your world beautiful, even if you aren't leaving the house today.

List seven things. Make a list of seven tasks that you do every week. Create your own form by making two columns on a piece of paper, labeled "Task" and "Upgrade." List one item for each day of the week. For example, your list might include driving, cooking, doing laundry, writing e-mails at work, mowing the lawn, talking on the phone, and paying bills.

Think of ways to upgrade. In the second column, write at least one way to make doing that task more enjoyable. Think of a really good way to do this, something that would make you look forward to engaging with this task. For example, if you listed "cook dinner," you might get excited about it by trying a new recipe, buying a new knife, or moving your CD player into the kitchen. Think about ways you can either upgrade the task by using nicer equipment or ways to enhance the environment while doing the task by implementing music or scents.

Be creative in making your tasks more fun and enjoyable. Make a shopping list and get everything you need for the week at one time. Give yourself a budget and go. Remember that many of the tasks you listed are things that you will be doing regularly—you should have an enjoyable, effective way of getting them done. You don't have to spend a lot of money to improve your experience, sometimes cleaning something or rearranging items that you use (for instance, a thorough cleaning of your refrigerator or reorganization of your desk drawer) will make things more enjoyable. As you go through your days, just keep asking yourself, "How can I make this more fun?"

Make It Better

Your day is filled with routine tasks. Take a moment to figure out how to make each and every one of them a little bit better, a little bit easier, and a little bit more fun.

Dealing with the Out-of-the-Ordinary with Grace and Style

We could all probably come up with amazingly optimized schedules and clever never-fail strategies for breezing through our days if every day was exactly the same as the day before. Unless you are in prison, however, this is probably far from your reality. Our ordinary days are peppered with unpredictable things—good and bad—that we have to work through: your child gets sick at school, your air conditioning stops working, your husband gets a raise (requiring a celebration), or your husband gets a bad performance review (requiring comforting). All of this is not directly related to your MS, but even this daily "noise" can have a huge impact on your symptoms and wellbeing as you try to juggle schedules, attention, and emotions.

As if that is not enough to contend with, interspersed into these days are life events and other occurrences and undertakings that range from mildly disruptive to monumental. There is the bad stuff that happens, the illnesses and deaths in the family, the layoffs and firings, the unexpected and undesirable job-related relocations. Then there are the good things, the things that make us smile, but also come with their own share of complicated logistics, high emotions, and general disruption. These things might include long-awaited and eagerly-anticipated voyages to exotic new places, beautiful weddings, once-in-a-lifetime career opportunities, and the biggie of long-term life-changers—a baby, or babies.

Unfortunately, there are no handy tips that I can give you that can make raising a child or moving your household a stress-free walk in the park. There are certain strategies, however, for getting through life that may come in handy, especially for those of us with MS who have found (or are still searching for) a fragile state of homeostasis and wellbeing that we are trying to preserve in the face of both gentle intrusions and potential earthquakes.

Make the routine stuff automatic. Put some real effort into getting yourself and your life organized in a way that makes sense to you. Do things that you do every day the same way every time. This could free up huge amounts of time and mental energy that you could use on the unexpected things or planning for larger events.

Take Charge

Your MS is constantly changing. Take control of what you can by making your environment and routine more consistent. Set up systems and methods for as many things as possible. Get organized and make things easier.

Reduce your decision burden. Let's say something that you are happy about is coming up—you are going on vacation, for instance. That is great, but even exciting, wonderful times are still full of obligations, such as physical needs, that must be met in order to keep going. This is especially true for those of us with MS, who can't always play it by ear in terms of schedules and activity levels. We might need to work in injections and regular rest periods. Whereas other people can say things such as, "I guess we might be able to find a taxi to maybe get us back up the mountain to our hotel," people with MS can't always take chances and may need to know exactly how they are going to get from one place to another before embarking on the adventure.

Make It Better

It takes extra effort for our MS brains to make decisions and process information, so remove unnecessary decisions and information from your world. This will result in less fatigue and help conserve precious energy.

Here is what I suggest you do. Sit quietly and visualize yourself on this vacation. See yourself packing your suitcase the night before. Imagine putting it in the car and going to the airport, checking in, and going through security . . . oops, gotta pull your syringes out of your carry-on with a prescription tag attached (and a note from your doc if you want to play it extra safe). Keep going to your gate—better make sure to check and see how far away it is and have the information on how to get a ride on one of those carts . . . .

Okay, you get the message. There are a million teeny steps involved in everything we do, and when you are trying to do things that don't happen every day, even one of these steps can be a huge obstacle if you aren't expecting it. In our example above, ideally you would have a pad of paper and write down all the things that you think of during your visualization. To be really strategic, you would keep going with the planning, learning about the place that you are going so well that you really don't have to make many decisions once you get there. Plan an itinerary, even including specific times and restaurants. Make reservations and buy tickets to give yourself "anchors." Even if you stray from your plans, you will have a point to return to, rather than finding yourself somewhere far from food at 3:00 in the afternoon and realizing you didn't have lunch and don't know how to get back to the hotel.

To some extent, this type of planning helps in all situations. When I was expecting my twins, I was so consumed with the discomforts and the difficulties of the pregnancy that the idea of taking care of actual infants seemed far away and pretty theoretical. I ended up with the prize of two healthy babies, but without having given much thought to my daily routine of diapers and bottles. As a result, nothing was really ready except two cribs and some cute flowers decorating the nursery wall. If I had taken the time to think through the things that I knew had to happen, I could have saved a great deal of emotional and physical stress and just ended up exhausted rather than exhausted *and* in a perpetual panic.

Maintain Maximum Independence in the Long Term

Certain animals are often referred to as "dignified." Take the bald eagle, for instance. A bald eagle is probably one of the most impressive animals on the planet. As flying creatures, they are literally above it all. They don't really appear to be worried about much of anything as they gaze around with those clear eyes looking for a small, scurrying (undignified) rodent to kill and eat.

The Real World

You can maintain your dignity even if you need help doing things.

Bad stuff happens to bald eagles, too. Several years ago, I visited the Alaska Raptor Rehabilitation Center in Sitka, Alaska. This facility was home to a variety of birds of prey that had fallen on bad times. Owls, falcons, hawks, and eagles that had been injured in some way (most often, it seemed, by slingshots or guns in the hands of young boys) were brought here to recuperate. If they recovered to the point of being able to live in the wild, they were released. If their injuries were so severe that the birds would not be able to function enough to fend for themselves, they would be kept at the center in very large enclosed areas.

One resident was Volta. Volta was a bald eagle who had flown into some power lines. During his recovery, it was discovered that he had an injury to a wing that limited his ability to fly.

Although Volta could not fly any long distance and could not fend for himself, he was one badass animal. Here was the definition of "dignity," embodied in a disabled eagle that needed help to get his basic needs met.

So, what does that have to do with the fact that we might need help doing all sorts of things that people with healthy myelin breeze through, things that even three-year-olds have mastered? It's about sense of self, it's about not letting the malfunctioning body parts define us or harm the essence of who we are. Often, taking a cold, hard look at what is really happening and what types of assistance are needed is what is required to keep us whole.

For example, imagine two women with noticeable, severe intention tremor that prevents them from successfully manipulating buttons or applying makeup and has led to frustration and embarrassment in social situations. One woman interprets this as a cue that this is *it*, the beginning of her downward decline into being a "disabled person," but she fiercely clings to her idea of independence, refusing any help and getting angry when it is offered. A formerly impeccable dresser to whom clothes and outward appearances were important, she resorts to wearing housecoats and t-shirts and avoids looking at herself in the mirror. Her social encounters become limited, then pretty much stop as she withdraws into herself. She simply doesn't feel good about herself. Conversely, the other woman in our example takes a deep breath, then looks at her wardrobe. Some buttons can be replaced with hidden Velcro, so that she can continue wearing her favorite things. She finds a lighter shade of lipstick and learns to apply it by resting her elbow on the counter, then moving her mouth over the lipstick, which she decides is pretty damn clever. She kisses her husband on the forehead as he helps her with tricky zippers and earrings, and leans more heavily on his arm than she used to. She thinks to herself that life is different, harder in many ways. However, life is still good and worth the effort—worth the fight, she muses as she looks outward toward the future.

Prioritize Your Priorities

As the mother of young children, I am witnessing firsthand the powerful human need for independence. I watch with amazement, usually having to restrain myself from intervening, as my girls try repeatedly to do "big girl" stuff—help me mix cookie batter, put on their own shoes, use a word correctly—often snarling something about "do it *myself*, Mommy." At the very same time, in my own body, I acutely feel the necessity of getting a little more help with things, just to make it through the day and accomplish the same things that fully-myelinated people do without a second thought. Especially at my peak fatigue times, I have often thought it would be a luxury to be treated like a three-year-old again, told what to do, fed, bathed, cuddled, and put to bed.

By the time many of us get diagnosed with MS and gradually begin needing help with things, however, we have already determined the best ways to do things, at least the ways that make the most sense to us. Subconsciously or not, we express who we are in the manner that we negotiate daily life—it's in the way that we hold our coffee cups, the brand of paper towels that we buy, the jobs that we hold and how we approach them, the choices we make about what to do with our finances.

When there comes a time that we cannot do it all—either for a short time or for the foreseeable future—we can take the opportunity to evaluate our situation to decide which things only we know how to do the "right way" and which things we would rejoice in seeing done by other people. Then we figure out how this can happen—where we need to compromise and where we don't.

Don't Panic

Needing physical help is only one kind of dependence, which doesn't mean that you need to give up who *you* are. You are in control and can be emotionally and socially independent, despite disability.

For instance, I have pretty much stopped driving and rely almost entirely on my husband to drive me around to run most errands, or just have him do them himself. This works fine for the most part, but initially meant that I lost control over the specifics of groceries. I love to cook and am a self-proclaimed "foodie," meaning that food is more than simple fuel—what comes out of my kitchen is an expression of who I am. Sending my poor husband for groceries was unfair to both of us (mostly him). Of course, I could write out a list and he would get those items on the list, but specifying brands and degrees of ripeness that I required began to try his patience. I would go about my unpacking the groceries with trepidation and use the "subpar" ingredients at my disposal with resignation and suffering. Nothing was *right* until I found a grocery store with a complementary "personal shopper," who was actually thrilled to have the specifics laid out to the point that I actually get calls to discuss the size of the Napa cabbages or the color of icing on shortbread cookies to make sure that I get just what I want.

When I can take a rare objective look at my pissiness regarding the groceries, I can say that a big part of those feelings had to do with not feeling normal, being unable to do my own damn grocery shopping, which I would inevitably extrapolate to being a loser of a wife and an unfit mother. Bottom line: I was pissed off that I had MS and that anger snuck out in fits over the wrong kind of extra virgin olive oil coming into my home. Whatever. Feelings are feelings and perception is reality, so I fixed the problem and moved on without too much embarrassing self-examination. Luckily, I am not as concerned about the minute details of the rest of the things that need to get done, and I am just happy that the household is running. Whether it is me doing things sloppily or my husband doing things differently than I would, so be it.

Mobility and Self-Care Independence

This is the big one, isn't it? It is one thing to wish that you could remodel a room, but need a little help with painting the crown molding because of balance issues. It is another matter altogether when you begin to get nervous about getting in and out of the bathtub when no one is home. Moving along the continuum from needing to hold your spouse's elbow, to using a cane, then a walker, then easing yourself into a wheelchair or a scooter, may require that we go through a mini grieving process at each concession that we make, at each new piece of equipment that we need.

I have read many useful and valuable things about approaching worsening disability with different attitudes in order to stay emotionally healthy, such as thinking of the increased reliance on mobility aids as a "transition" rather than a "loss," or to be proud that you are taking steps to address a problem, rather than living in a state of denial. Regardless of how you get your head around the problem, there will undoubtedly be times that you watch others traipse along *sans* walker or talk about a vacation where they climbed hundreds of stairs to enjoy a spectacular view of the city from the belltower of a church, and think, "Why me?" Go ahead—indulge yourself in these thoughts for a little while. Then move on to "Okay, what now?" and look at your situation from a strategic angle.

There are people that are skilled and ready to work with you to optimize your abilities. Physical therapists (PTs) can help you with getting the most out of your body in terms of improving balance, gait, strength, and flexibility. Occupational therapists (OTs) are trained to help you function better in the world, both by helping you do tasks more efficiently from an energy standpoint, as well as adapting your environment to make things easier by modifying living and work spaces with things like grip bars and modifications to your car. They also help with mobility devices, like walkers and scooters. The PT and OT may work together with you to make sure that you are using your assistive and mobility aids correctly and getting the most benefit from them without wasting precious energy. Your doctor can help you figure out whom you need to see and write necessary orders and prescriptions for therapy.

Financial Independence

I really don't like budgeting. I am the kind of person who will get all excited about a subscription or service, saying, "But it's only 80 dollars a month!" and be stunned and dismayed when my husband shows me how that seemingly-reasonable amount magically transforms into an annual cost of almost a thousand dollars. Regardless of how you feel about budgets, it is a really, *really* good idea to figure out what your situation is and what your financial future might hold.

Discussing this in detail is beyond the scope of the book (and my fiscal acumen), but what I would recommend is visiting with a qualified financial planner who could help you figure out where you stand and what your goals should be, as well as steps to take to get there. You can start your education with a book jointly produced by the National MS Society, the Paralyzed Veterans of America, and the National Endowment for Financial Education, titled *Adapting: Financial Planning for a Life with Multiple Sclerosis*. This 72-page book covers all aspects of the impact that MS might have on your finances, including health insurance considerations and estate planning, as well as helpful worksheets, spreadsheets, and checklists for figuring it all out. It can be downloaded for free from the NMSS Web site (enter "financial planning" into the search box) or by calling 800-667-7131 to request that a free copy be mailed to you. The MS Society also has a program called "Money Matters" to provide expertise to individuals with MS, both for people needing immediate financial advice, as well as those who are planning for the future.

Workplace Independence

Perhaps not surprisingly (although I *was* actually kind of surprised by these statistics when I first heard them), given the nature of multiple sclerosis, the majority of MSers in the United States are unemployed— an estimated 55 to 65 percent of us no longer hold paying jobs. It also seems that the longer people live with MS, the more likely they are to leave the workplace—more specifically, an estimated 70 to 80 percent of people who have been living with an MS diagnosis for more than 15 years fall into this category.[1]

What many "experts" cannot figure out is *why* exactly this is. Of course, the first thought of researchers was that people with MS become increasingly disabled and physically can't stand the rigors of holding down a full-time position. However, people smarter than I on this topic have turned it upside-down and inside-out and have concluded that physical and cognitive limitations only explain some of what is happening, as 75 percent of unemployed people left their positions voluntarily and 80 percent say they are still able to work. Researchers bring up other factors as playing a part, such as discrimination and other workplace variables, as well as work disincentives in both private disability insurance and programs of the Social Security Administration. I guess the very most interesting statistic here from my point of view is that three-quarters of the currently unemployed people with MS actually want to go back to work.

Rosalind Joffe, coauthor of *Keep Working, Girlfriend: Navigating the Workplace with an Autoimmune Disease*, insists that people with chronic diseases can benefit greatly from staying in (or reentering) the workplace, despite some of the extra challenges. A person living with MS herself, she cites many benefits to "staying in the game," which include things like reduced poverty, improved quality of life and better health, and an increased sense of achievement and power over one's illness.[2]

I, of course, have my own thoughts about this subject, which hits a little close to home. There are shades of gray in the idea of "too disabled" to hold down a job. I know that I could function as well as many other people in a normal full-time employment situation—all the time outside of the actual work hours, however, would be spent either resting up for the job or recovering from the hours that I just put in, including a nap over my lunch hour. In a situation where I can make my own schedule, such as with writing or some of the consulting work that I have done, I can almost double my productive hours in a day by resting when I need to and being able to mentally shut down and perform routine tasks or isolate myself from others (rather than mustering for meetings) for long periods. I know that not everyone can work like this or has the opportunity to earn money outside the traditional office or other work settings. I just don't think even the most well-designed research surveys can capture all of the factors that constitute a decision to leave the workplace.

If you have left your job or are in the process of making this decision, make sure it is not a hasty one. Do not scrawl out your resignation letter in the throes of Solu-Medrol-induced anxiety or immediately after arriving home following the appointment where you receive your MS diagnosis. Think it through. Make a list of the pros and cons. Spend some time with a financial planner. Visualize what it will be like to be home alone day after day. Picture yourself five and ten years from now and think about what you will be doing, rather than focusing on how boring certain parts of your job might be or how annoying some of your colleagues are.

As it turns out, many people with MS *do* stay employed in traditional jobs for various reasons. You know what your reasons might be—you might love your job or you might hate it, you might feel great or you might feel terrible most of the time, you might see a chance for career advancement that makes you feel hopeful or you might be treading water. Then there is the question of very simple economics—work equals money, which most of us need to get by.

As people with MS, in many situations we have the Incredible Hulk on our side as far as workplace rights go, in the form of the Americans with Disabilities Act (ADA). The ADA basically guarantees that people with disabilities have equal rights in society, which includes workplace and educational settings (among other things). It is a mighty piece of legislation that not only says that it is to the benefit of society to keep people with disabilities productive and active, but backs this up with the mandate to provide reasonable accommodations to employees with disabilities to perform the essential functions needed in their jobs. Though the law is wonderful, it is important to understand its parameters.

One thing that has been controversial and problematic with the original ADA is the definition of "disabled."[3] The original law was intentionally written in broad language in regards to who was protected, mostly focusing on the idea that discrimination for pretty much *any* reason was wrong. Over the years, however, the definition of "disabled" has become more and more narrow and has excluded many people with manageable conditions (meaning that symptoms could be controlled, such as with diabetes, epilepsy, and cancer). This meant that people with MS who were doing well on disease-modifying drugs or coping with their symptoms using medications and other methods were not covered. The implications for people with MS were terrible— there is no need to review the entire list of invisible symptoms that many of us grapple with, and it is folly to think that a symptom that is "managed" brings a person back up to the physical level of a healthy person. I shudder to imagine the nightmare of trying to describe MS-related fatigue, neuropathic pain, or cognitive dysfunction to an unsympathetic employer, especially for the MSer that has no accompanying mobility problems or other visible symptoms. I imagine this is why many of the aforementioned people left the workplace.

Fortunately, disability rights activists, including many people with MS have successfully restored lost power to the ADA. In September 2008, President Bush signed the ADA Amendments Act (formerly known as the ADA Restoration Act), which became effective January 1, 2009. This amendment basically reinstates the intended protections, as it says that it doesn't matter if the condition or symptom can be made better or controlled by medication, it doesn't matter if it comes and goes, and it doesn't have to severely restrict major life activities to be considered a "disability."

There are a couple of other restrictions on the ADA. As far as the workplace goes, it only applies to companies with at least 15 employees. Secondly, the law calls for "reasonable accommodations," which means that any adaptations to your work environment or schedule will not cause the employer too much money or disrupt things a great deal (aka "undue hardship"). Lastly, you must be able to perform the parts of your job that are necessary to that position—the standards of the job description stay the same.

You can find out much more about the ADA and your workplace rights by starting with the Job Accommodations Network (JAN), found at www.jan.wvu.edu, which is run by the U.S. Department of Labor's Office of Disability Employment Policy. It has comprehensive information about specific protections under the ADA, as well as resources such as employer trainings, information regarding employer tax incentives, and specific suggestions in terms of adaptive measures for the workplace. You can also find information specific to people with MS by looking on the website of the NMSS or talking to someone at your local chapter. If things at work do not go as smoothly as you think they should, meaning that you think your employer or others in your work environment are not complying with the provisions of the ADA, you can file a complaint with the U.S. Equal Employment Opportunity Commission/EEOC (www.eeoc.gov). This, however, should be used as a last resort, as it can get ugly. I recommend talking things through with your employer first—I know people who have sued their employers for various reasons and the results have been a mixed bag. They may have kept their jobs, but they often end up lonely, isolated, and the target of anger and hostility—and they often end up quitting anyway. Although laws can protect us in many ways, they cannot control a person's emotions and how socially "warm" and "fuzzy" (or not) our environment is.

Long-Term Care

In the past, when I thought about long-term care, my mind immediately conjured up a vision of a poorly-run nursing home embroiled in legal battles around elder neglect. Fortunately, that is *not* what long-term care is about, and finding out more about different long-term care options makes the whole subject much less scary. There are several options to meet the needs of people with different levels of disability and caretaking situations. You might be surprised to know that having someone help in your home, either on a consistent basis or occasionally to provide respite care so that your family caretakers can have a break, falls into this category. There are also residential options, called "assisted living residences" that are designed to keep people in their own apartment while providing services to keep them safe and engaged. These programs often include meals, social events, exercise classes, maid services, as well as monitoring and emergency call systems. Then there is the more traditional nursing home option, which provides round-the-clock care for residents. Services vary by location, but your local chapter of the MS Society can tell you not only what is available, but which services are the most appropriate for people with MS in your situation. Also, MSF Home Care Assistance Grant Program helps link up people with MS to appropriate local services. (See "Find and use resources for people with MS" in Chapter 11 for more information.)

Power of Attorney and Advance Directives

It may seem paradoxical to include these things in a section about maintaining independence, but it is actually something that you can do to ensure that your wishes are heard and decisions are made as you would want them to be. If done right, these measures keep you in control of your situation. A "power of attorney" designates a specific person (your "agent") of your choosing to make decisions on your behalf. There are many permutations of powers of attorney, which include those that kick in only during a remission (limited power of attorney), those that only apply to health care decisions (durable power of attorney for health care, medical directive, health care proxy), those that are effective immediately, and those that are effective on a specified date. Then there are those that are "general," meaning you give your agents all the power to do anything in your name. It is important that you execute these correctly and choose the right type for your situation. So important, in fact, that I am going to refrain from saying much more besides "talk to an attorney." Your local chapter of the MS Society will probably have a list of lawyers in your area who have experience with issues around MS, and may even have some that are willing to work with you on a pro-bono (free) basis.

The Real World

No one likes planning for the worst. Do it anyway. It is respectful to those who love you.

The Bottom Line

The idea of control is a funny thing. Take, for instance, the swine flu scares of early 2009. People were panicked because there wasn't a vaccine available yet. Many of these same people, however, skip the yearly flu shot against the much-deadlier influenza that kills over 35,000 people annually. I guess that people want the decision regarding whether or not to take precautions to be *their* decision, rather feeling a lack of control because there are no options available to them.

Take Charge

Don't overlook opportunities that allow you to be in control. Make the effort to control what you can in your world and don't let things slide.

It is true that, as people living with MS, certain things are out of our control. We do not know if we will feel good enough or even be physically able to do something that we want to do. Considering what will happen long-term is difficult, but even trying to make plans for later the same day can be pretty impossible for many of us. That said, there are things that we can influence if we approach life rationally and strategically. We can prepare for unanticipated relapses or symptom worsening so that our attention can be turned to dealing with our very immediate physical reality (either temporary or more permanent), while the things that usually require our attention are taken care of by others. We can learn to identify our stressors and separate our emotions from the reality of what is happening. We can make the things that we have to do on a regular basis not contribute to stress, but work to make them more enjoyable.

We can figure out what it is that constitutes the essence of us and patch together solutions to preserve that unique core of ourselves even as the world swirls around us and our bodies continue to change.

8

Create Health in New Places

Whenever I am asked about my health or how I am feeling, I immediately do a little MS symptom "inventory." If I am feeling better than I did yesterday, I am "healthier." On the other hand, if my symptoms seem a little, or a lot, worse—my fatigue is slowing me down more, the tingling in my feet is a little more pronounced, my MS hug is "huggier"—clearly (in my mind), my health is going downhill.

It is a shame to think in such an MS-centric way, especially because the official definition of health is "a state of complete physical, mental, and social well-being and not merely the absence of disease or infirmity."[1] This is the definition that has been used by the World Health Organization since 1948.

Do Your Best

Just like you are more than your MS, your health is more than your MS symptoms. Don't neglect your overall health by getting lost in your MS.

Don't feel bad if, like me, you focus on your MS, or any immediate discomfort you may have—a cold or a bout of nausea—when thinking about your health. Most people do not think about their health until something is physically wrong; health is something they either have or do not have. But when you really think about it, this understanding of health doesn't work for all, or even most, circumstances. Think about a young person who is physically healthy—strong, in great shape—but suffers from depression. Then consider someone with a debilitating illness, who has a rich spiritual life, enjoys a strong social support net-work, interacts with loved ones, and takes time to appreciate fine food, literature, and music. Who is healthier? Who "feels" better?

It is often shocking to me when I go to the doctor to find out that I have a non-MS problem that needs attention, because that seems a little unfair. Fair or not, it is true that people with MS are subject to the same health problems, as a result of aging or lifestyle choices, as the rest of the world. On the other hand, we also have some of the same opportunities to increase our health, as well.

Humans are complex creatures, and there is far more to overall health than physical functioning. Granted, when we don't feel good physically, it is hard to feel healthy. However, by putting effort into examining other aspects of health, including social health, spiritual health, and mental health, it is easier to not only put physical ailments into perspective, but also to make changes to habits that could help us feel better in general. Illnesses may change priorities and strengthen relationships. True health encompasses our bodies, our emotions, our minds, our relationships, our homes, our behaviors, and our spiritual selves. Each day you can make gains, even if your symptoms are worsening.

Physical health. Clearly, when we feel bad, it is hard to feel "healthy," period; however, as mentioned (and as will be discussed in the second half of this chapter), physical health is more than MS and its symp-toms. It's also true that if there is something you can do to improve your physical wellbeing, you will probably feel better overall, which may include a reduction in your MS symptoms.

Just think of all the things that you could do today to feel better. You could exercise; add one serving of vegetables to your lunch or din-ner; have your last cup of coffee before 3 pm, so that you can go to bed 45 minutes earlier; or anything else to make incremental changes to your well-being.

Emotional health. The emotional aspect of health, whether a person is living with MS or not, is often overlooked until constant stress mani-fests itself as a physical problem—headaches, gastrointestinal prob-lems, and (yes), many MS symptoms can be made much worse by neglecting emotional health. "Emotional health" seems like such a vague term that it is difficult to sum it up in a simple definition. It is not about being happy all the time, and it doesn't mean that you are grateful for every minute of every day as some people claim, (usually after a horrible tragedy has befallen them, but from which they have either healed or escaped). Instead, it means that you are strong enough to weather what life sends your way, letting some of the bad stuff roll off your back and grabbing the opportunity to enjoy the good stuff. These things describe people who are emotionally healthy: they are content, they laugh often and have fun, they are able to find and nurture fulfilling relationships, they can effectively balance work and other activities with rest and relaxation, they are able to deal with stress, and they can adapt to both planned and unexpected changes. In addition, emotionally healthy people have self-confidence and high self-esteem.

Social health. I know this is important, and I can describe someone who is socially healthy and someone who needs help in this area, but when I tried to pull together a definition that covered these ideas, I was stumped. After researching this topic, I found this definition of "social health": "that dimension of an individual's well-being that concerns how he gets along with other people, how other people react to him, and how he interacts with social institutions and societal mores."[2] Research has shown that people who are socially involved with their communities recover faster from illnesses and are less affected by symptoms or disabilities.

Look, I confess that there are days that I glare at my telephone whenever it rings. During these times, I resent anyone who sends me an e-mail to see how I am doing or if I would like to get together—if the message contains emoticons of little winking smiley faces or extra exclamation points, I might sink into a pit of disdainful planning to become a complete recluse. These are the moments that I cling to my armor of "nobody understands what this feels like" in order to make the whole darn MS mess go away. Guess what? It hasn't worked yet. I have found that the pissier and less social I am, the worse I feel. I have also found that whenever I muster the energy to go to a party that I had wasted a week dreading, or actually go through all of the steps it takes (really hard things like showering, brushing my teeth, and finding a clean shirt) to go out with another person, most of the time I end up enjoying myself. Not only that, but I forget about my MS or my *symptôme du jour* for that time, as my energy is focused on someone or something else for a little while.

That said, it is also important that people with MS connect with others who are going through the same thing. Only someone else with MS-related fatigue can understand that horror in a few words. Getting cheered on by others with MS for some progress you made against a symptom also has a very, very special quality—emoticons and a profusion of exclamation points are extremely welcome in these circumstances, as in "A whole night without getting up to pee?!?!?! You go, girl!!! ;.)"

Intellectual health. Intellectual health, in my opinion, is characterized by the ability to fluidly think thoughts that incorporate creativity, common sense, and knowledge gained from books and through living. It is the ease with which these aspects of cognition come together in a coherent and appropriate way.

To understand what it is like to experience a lack of intellectual health, think back to when you may have watched five straight hours of *Green Acres* or *Happy Days* reruns. By the end of the television marathon, you feel slower, kind of dazed, drained of energy, and lacking the motivation to do much of anything besides eat Cheetos. On the other hand, when you have an intellectually "snappy" kind of day, you get stimulating little mini-rushes of happiness from little endorphin releases in your brain—this might come after giving a good presentation at work, listening to a reading at a bookstore, holding your own in a fast-paced and interesting conversation, or finishing a challenging crossword puzzle.

When it comes to maintaining intellectual health, the mantra "use it or lose it" is truly appropriate (although, admittedly, a little annoying). Your brain *needs* stimulation to perform well in executive functioning. For those of us living with multiple sclerosis, this is crucial, as many of us feel like we are "swimming upstream" intellectually in our fight against MS-related cognitive dysfunction. Cognitive dysfunction as a symptom of MS manifests in several ways, including: problems organizing thoughts, short-term memory deficits, distractibility and attention difficulties, word-finding problems, and slower speed of information processing. Here is the good news, folks: it is all still there, it just takes a little extra time and effort to get to it ("it" being our intellect, our smarts, ourselves).

So, do things to improve your intellectual health. Read a book—better yet, join a book club; listen to a podcast instead of music while you are driving; take a class to learn a foreign language; master a new computer program; do a crossword puzzle; pick an issue that you are interested in and research it on the Internet; attend a lecture at the local library or university; watch a foreign-language movie with subtitles, then discuss it with someone. In other words, keep your brain active.

Healthy surroundings. Look around you right now. Assuming that you are at home, and not reading this book on a subway, in a mall, or on an airplane, you should be able to find a calm place to rest your eyes. Your ears should be soothed by the sounds of silence, nature, or (maybe) tranquil music—if you do hear other people, such as your children, it should be happy sounds of soft laughter and conversation floating to your ears. You shouldn't notice any smells, aside from the occasional light scent of fresh-cut grass drifting in your open window.

Okay, seriously. How far does this deviate from your reality? How sad does that make you? Your home should be a lovely retreat where you can relax and recharge, but most of us probably spend a great deal of mental energy "shutting out" the stress-inducing aspects of our home. Think about what you can do to make at least a small corner of your home more closely resemble a spa-like escape from the outside world—both today (turn off the TV and light a candle) and in the future (paint a room in earth tones and soften the lighting).

Spiritual health. I was unhappy with the definitions that I could find of "spiritual health" or "spirituality," as they all fairly quickly veered down different paths of specific religions or beliefs. Although that is where most of us will end up when we think about what these words mean to us, putting out any definition from a specific set of beliefs can only result in excluding some valid ideas about spirituality. So, left to my own devices, I am going to define spiritual health as the well-being of the soul, that part of a person that is intangible. I am going to leave the exact meaning of "soul" up to each of you. For some people, the soul is an immortal spirit that temporarily inhabits our physical bodies before moving onto another body when we die. For others, it is the essence of a person that is basically the sum of who a person is, comprised of thoughts, feelings, actions—a personality. Then there are a whole bunch of other definitions in the middle of this spectrum, or on other spectra altogether. Regardless of your take on the matter, it is pretty hard to argue that spiritual health is not important.

To give your spiritual health a boost, try making a gratitude list of all the things (people, places, experiences, books, art, food, basically anything that makes you happy) in your life that you are grateful for and adding one item to it every day; attending a religious worship service of your choice; praying at a set time every day; or even just going to a place that inspires you, such as the forest, an art museum, a field of flowers, or a cemetery where a relative is buried.

Tips for Creating Health in New Places:

Be creative. Think of anything you can do that makes your life better or makes you feel good. Have crazy ideas. Don't limit yourself because of time, money, or other obstacles. Any idea you might have can be broken down into steps. If some of your ideas can't really happen right away, like taking a vacation or getting a dog, you can get books to research different resorts that you might like to visit or plan to go to a local dog show to start investigating the different breeds of dogs that might be right for you. Actively thinking about nice things can contribute to health in immeasurable ways.

But do try some things that are within reach. When choosing activities to do, make sure you do include some small things that you can accomplish in a day or two. Maybe you'll begin by cleaning up some clutter in your house, or even just clearing the magazines off of the coffee table. Maybe you'll finally get the oil changed in your car so you don't have to think about that anymore. Go to the farmers' market and try a new kind of leafy green vegetable. Health can be found anywhere.

Keep searching for ideas to expand health. Go on a health scavenger hunt throughout the day. Can you make changes to your environment, how you do things, or with whom you do them that will add health to your life?

Do Your Best
Really push yourself to find more health in new places. Do everything you can.

Offset negative thoughts with positive ideas. Try to invest the same amount of time, emotion, and energy into improving your health as you spend thinking about your MS. Every time you worry about a symptom worsening or your long-term prospects, balance that by taking an action to improve your health somewhere. Use your emotional concerns as cues for you to focus on your overall health.

Your Physical Health Is More than Your MS

As I mentioned, many of us with MS think of our physical health in terms of the symptoms that we have. We start with the notion of a flawed body and concentrate on those flaws, rather than thinking about what we can do to feel better.

Thinking about physical wellness in my MS-burdened self reminds me of my experience of buying a "perfect" house. I was buoyed by fantasies about family meals and romantic moments and laughing babies in my new home; however, when the home inspection was handed over it burst that little fantasy bubble as it enumerated all of the problems with my soon-to-be new house. It contained items as trivial as leaky faucets and as big as foundation flaws; the accompanying pictures showed details of mold, mildew, rot, possible termite damage, faulty building practices, and places where corners were cut. From that moment on, even years later, I still look at the personal touches and the love that I have put into this house and occasionally still see my efforts as icing on top of flaws. Even when everything is clean and organized and the details are just right, gone is my giddy vision of the perfect house.

It's hard to learn not to think of our bodies that way; at least it was for me. I would put the effort in to work out, to eat better, to really take care of myself, then I would remember that I had trouble spelling a word that morning or that I had areas of lipoatrophy on my thighs. These realizations took away from the progress that I had made and reminded me that I would never be perfect, no matter how much I worked at it. It took me much longer than it should have to realize that I should not aim for perfection in pursuing health and wellness, because that is a certain prescription for failure; however, the goal of "doing better" in my habits and how I take care of myself is a noble—and doable—one.

Having multiple sclerosis has little impact on overall life expectancy in most cases. For the most part, people with MS live with the same guidelines and suggestions about healthy aging as everyone else does. You know, the basic, common sense things like to live a long and healthy life you have to take care of your heart, your brain, and the rest of your body.

As people with MS, we have extra responsibility when it comes to taking care of our bodies. Most of us MSers are especially aware that it is crucial to keep ourselves as healthy as possible in order to keep on functioning well.

Strive for Better

I am going to share with you my philosophy for keeping the body going without getting despondent, obsessed or caught up in circular debates about what is the "right" approach to healthy living: *strive for a little better every day*. That's it, that's all there is to it, but it took me a long time to get here.

Do Your Best

Do everything possible to make today a tiny bit "healthier" than yesterday. Regardless of your MS situation, there is a lot of health out there for you to grab.

What do I mean by "strive for a little better every day?" It's very simple. We know on a fundamental level what healthy choices look like—easy things, like grapes instead of a Twinkie, a little yoga instead of that third hour of a video game, sleeping instead of doodling around on the Internet at 3:00 am—things like that. Yet, in many, maybe most, cases we reject those choices because we like to have a concrete strategy, with specific steps and instructions, rather than relying on our own instincts. We wait to start improving our habits until we find the perfect plan, then we make it an "all or nothing" endeavor. But it is precisely because the program for the "right way to live" often involves complicated exercise programs and diet plans that we fail to meet most of the objectives that we had at the beginning of these endeavors. Then we let things slip even more.

Let's start fresh. Let's see what we can do to make the most of what we've got, but still have a good time and maintain our sense of self, and humor, while doing so. Let's tune in a little better to what our bodies and minds instinctively know and take it from there.

With these instructions in mind, there are some fundamental things that we need to do for our physical selves to stay healthy. While striving for a little better each day, we need to: eat (fuel our bodies), get some form of exercise (move our bodies), sleep (rest our bodies), de-stress and relax (restore our bodies), and get things checked out on occasion (maintain our bodies).

Fuel Your Body

You will be disappointed if you have flipped to this section hoping to see a recommendation for a specific diet that will help you recover from MS symptoms or slow the progression of your MS. Mostly I just want to talk to you about making wise choices about what you put into your body, then turn the project over to you.

It is true to say that most people do not have an excellent understanding of nutrition and have not mastered a list of what is healthy and what is not. How could they when there is so much contradictory advice being thrown around? We are told to eat more fish, for example, only to encounter reams of information about toxic mercury content, unsafe fish farming practices, certain species of fish forced onto the endangered species list, and inappropriate antibiotic use in fish. We are told at the same time that eggs are both bad for you and good for you. And I am pretty sure that more than a few social occasions have been ruined by overly zealous people getting into the low-carb vs. low-fat debate.

All of that aside, most of us have the basic knowledge and instincts to be able to eat in a way that does not harm us. Although I don't claim to know of a universal food plan that will make everyone that follows it feel better, there are a couple of things that we can do to eat so that we don't feel worse, and that would be a huge improvement indeed for many people.

Cultivate good eating habits. Although what we eat is clearly important, *how* we eat is often the culprit in overeating and making poor food choices. Many of us stuff food in while sitting in front of the TV, messing around on the computer, driving our cars, or doing any number of things that distract us from exactly what and how much is going in our mouths. Here are a couple of things to experiment with to bring this under control, and make eating a more mindful (and dignified) activity:

only eat while sitting at a table; when you eat, eat—don't multitask; try putting your fork down between bites and focus on the food that you are chewing.

Do Your Best

Eat to feel physically good 15 minutes after you stop eating. Eat for your body.

Just saying . . . Okay, I don't want to spew a bunch of rules, but there are a couple of truisms that it never hurts to be reminded of. Michael Pollan, author of *In Defense of Food: An Eater's Manifesto*, implores us to "Eat food. Not too much. Mostly plants."[3] This pretty much sums it up, especially if you are a little thoughtful in your definition of "food," to the exclusion of things that are made entirely in laboratories or that in no way resemble anything that people ate a century ago.

Do Your Best

"Eat food. Not too much. Mostly plants."—Michael Pollan

Consider the possibility of food sensitivities. There are people who claim that we can cure, or at least recover from MS and its symptoms by paying attention to what we eat, namely eliminating things that our immune systems might be sensitive to. I'm not jumping into that debate right now, but I will tell you that food sensitivities can affect how you feel and how much your symptoms bother you. Through a little desperate experimentation, I discovered that gluten did not agree with me. I cut it out; I felt better. A couple years later, the same thing happened with legumes (beans and peanuts). As a result, I have a pretty limited diet, but it is worth it to feel even a little better. If you are interested, try eliminating suspect foods (gluten, legumes, milk, and soy are big culprits) for 2 weeks to see what happens, then do a "challenge" by eating a large amount. Trust me, you'll know if there is a problem. If you want to get serious about this, the best course of action is to see an allergist, who can perform specific blood or skin prick tests to give you more definitive answers.

Move Your Body

Study after study after study shows that exercise is critical to people with MS. It can improve fatigue, flexibility, stamina, and problems with spasticity, as well as symptoms of depression.

Do Your Best

Fatigue is a big part of MS. Get more energy by exercising. No, really—try it and see for yourself.

Figure out ways you can exercise and get physical activity without overheating and triggering the effects of MS-related heat intolerance. Focus on balance and flexibility. Your doctor can write you a prescription for physical therapy, which can help you build your muscles, improve balance, or move more efficiently. Ask trainers and instructors to help solve your problems. A good yoga instructor, for example, should be able to help customize a routine for your body.

The daily 15. By doing something physical every day, you can quickly build a daily habit of moving more. You can start by simply scheduling 15 minutes each day for activity. Over the course of a couple of weeks, you can gradually increase that time by 2 minutes every day pretty painlessly to get to 30 minutes and experiment with different types and intensities of physical activity. Your activity doesn't have to be traditional exercise—you can garden, do seated Tai Chi from a wheelchair, stretch—whatever gets your body moving.

Rest Your Body

You need to sleep. More specifically, you need to sleep between 7 and 9 hours each night. Unfortunately, many of us with MS have a very busy nocturnal schedule, which includes such activities as getting up dozens of times to urinate, paying attention to our willful spastic legs, tending to our restless legs syndrome, feeling our feet tingle, riding the Solu-Medrol insomnia and anxiety train, or lying there fretting about a new symptom or whether our insurance is going to cover a procedure. It's hard to fit sleep into that sort of agenda, which results in us getting very little quality sleep, thus compounding our already horrific fatigue.

The first thing to try, of course, is working with your doctor to address any symptom that is keeping you awake. Some of these can be treated effectively and easily with medications, and it is worth a try.

The next strategy involves various approaches to improving your "sleep hygiene." Sleep hygiene is overlooked, as most people think that sleep is something that your body should just be able to do, like breathing. In order to fall asleep fast and stay asleep, you may need to retrain your body. Here are some things to try:

Only use your bed for sleeping. If you read, watch TV, or even think in bed, you are telling your body that something other than sleep needs to be done. This is confusing to the primitive parts of our brain that control basic bodily functions like sleep. In order to retrain your body, you are going to have to send only one message each night: "It's time to sleep." What you are going to do is simple: wait until you are tired, then lie down and try to sleep. If you can't fall asleep within 15 minutes, get up and do something really boring and calming, and only use dim lights. Try to go to sleep again when you feel tired. For those of you who have been fretting since reading the heading of this paragraph, don't worry—sex is an approved bed activity that can help you sleep better.

Make It Better

Do everything possible to fix your sleep. Poor sleep makes everything worse.

Light and dark. This one is also pretty easy. Make sure that you are exposed to sunlight during the day and that you dim the lights as night approaches. The reasons for this are simple—what makes you fall asleep are changes in the level of the hormone melatonin circulating in your body. During the day, light stimulates a part of the brain, known as the *suprachiasmatic nucleus*, which tells the pineal gland to decrease the melatonin level when it is light out and to increase it when it is dark. The brighter the light, the bigger the decrease, and the darker the dark, the bigger the increase of melatonin.

Avoid sleep thieves. There are four of them: caffeine, alcohol, stress, and nicotine. Caffeine, which is a stimulant, keeps the body alert and energized. Your body can process 50% of a cup of coffee in 6 hours (the half-life of caffeine). This week, have no caffeine in the 6 hours before you go to sleep, including chocolate and tea. Using alcohol to fall asleep will keep you from having deep dream cycles of sleep, and will also cause blood sugar spikes at inconvenient times, both of which will wake you up. A glass of wine with dinner is fine if you are going to be up for a few more hours, as your body takes about an hour per drink to process the alcohol. That means if you want to drink two glasses of wine, you should be finished at least two hours before going to bed. Stress will interfere with your ability to fall asleep by sending a message to your brain that there is something important that you need to be doing other than sleeping. As for nicotine . . . Among other reasons to quit smoking, a study at Johns Hopkins showed that smokers are four times more likely to complain of poor sleep quality than non-smokers.[4]

Have a nightly ritual. Your body loves habits. By creating a habit that is strongly associated with sleep, your body will know exactly what to do when you lie down in bed. Decide what you would like to do during your ritual. Some people like to read in a comfortable chair for a few minutes. Other like to just stretch, brush their teeth, and be calm. A warm bath or shower can help get you into that relaxation zone. Changing the scent in your bedroom can also be very helpful, because your sense of smell is tightly linked to the emotional control centers of the brain. Like Pavlov's dog, you can train yourself to feel sleepy by simply smelling a certain smell when you are tired. Try lighting a scented candle or using a lavender-scented pillow or room spray. The important thing is to repeat the same ritual every night to establish cues that tell your body it is time to sleep.

Restore Your Body

Being stressed is unhealthy for anyone. It drains your energy, worsens your sleep, and damages your long-term health. It also looks like stress can lead to or worsen relapses.

There are several things you can do to reduce stress, but one of the easiest ones with instant benefits is meditation. In fact, most of the other stress-reducing techniques have a meditative component at their core: prayer, music therapy, art therapy, creative visualization, and even things like doing everyday tasks, such as folding laundry or preparing dinner, mindfully.

Meditation can reduce stress, decrease negative emotions, increase creativity, and promote good health, all while helping you live more mindfully and deliberately. You can also benefit from meditation if you are interested in establishing more control over your emotions, as well as cultivating your mental skills and increasing your ability to concentration.

Make It Better

Meditation is great for MS—it trains the brain to quiet down and focus. We could *all* (MS or not) use help with that.

Meditation is not about making your brain stop thinking—that is impossible. It's more about letting the "noise" die down by not engaging with the thoughts that come and letting them drift past. Give it a try.

Here's how to meditate:

Schedule a time. Schedule 5 minutes each day this week to sit and focus. This should be the same time every day. Make sure that you will not be interrupted by anything during this time—no phones and no knocks on the door.

Sit. Sit comfortably in an alert position. You can sit in a chair or on a cushion placed on the floor—it does not matter. Make your back as straight as possible. Keep your head level and look slightly downward. Pick one spot on the wall and stare at it. You intention is to only sit— so no looking around the room. If you want, you can close your eyes, but try not to fall asleep. Put your hands anywhere that is comfortable.

Focus. Choose one of the following to focus on:

- Pick a word that has some meaning to you, like "peace," "quiet," or "calm." Repeat that word slowly to yourself as you sit.
- Count your breaths. Every time you exhale, count. When you get to ten, return to one.

That's pretty much it. Try it a couple of times and experience the benefits for yourself.

Maintain Your Body

My neuro rolls his eyes and refers me to what he calls "real doctors" whenever I ask him about something health-related that is not directly linked to my central nervous system. He doesn't want to hear about (or think about) my cholesterol, my pap smears, my mammograms, my itchy skin, or my drips and sniffles. It's just not his territory.

For many of us, a doctor is a doctor is a doctor, and the map of our body and who "controls" each region is a little unclear. I think back with great love of my grandmother, sitting in her paper gown on the oncologist's exam table, with fire in her eyes and frustration in her voice as she tried to get the roles of her various physicians clarified. "I know you are in charge of these," she told the oncologist, pointing to her mastectomy scar and remaining breast, "but who in the hell do I need to talk to about this crap?!?" she spat, waving her hand over ankles uncomfortably swollen from a combination of medication side effects and failing circulation.

Unfortunately, MS doesn't give us a pass from all of the other stuff that comes along with being a human who is getting older. Although it doesn't quite seem fair, we still need to do all those things that other people do, or should do, to make sure that the rest of our body is doing its job. At the very least, all of us need to see a general practitioner (or family doc, or gynecologist, or internist) at least once a year, who will examine us, screen us, and direct us to specialists if needed. Oh, yeah, don't forget the dentist, too.

The Bottom Line

Take a minute and think of some of the people that you know. Let's start with that guy (we all know one of these) who has no physical disabilities, a stable financial situation, a family that seems to like each other well enough and are all healthy, and a nice house. Still, nothing is ever good enough; he is convinced that everything (including the weather and the economy) and everyone (including the president of the United States) are aligned specifically against *him*. He is, slowly but surely, accumulating all sorts of health problems from stress.

Then consider someone else you might know who lives with a much more challenging situation. I think of my dear, dear friend who I have known since the first day of kindergarten. Her 7-year-old son had a stroke at birth and is severely disabled, yet she tells me how lucky she is that he "only" has a couple of seizures a week. Her laugh sounds like a tinkling fountain as she proudly recounts his progress at pointing to a card with a picture of a cracker on it when he is hungry or drinking from a special cup with two handles. She is the embodiment of grace and an inspiration, yet she always tells me that I am wonderful and she is lucky to be my friend.

Which one do you want to know, and more importantly, who do you want to be?

9

Reform Relationships on Your Terms

I would like to think that I do not let my MS define me as a person. However, I have noticed something interesting—the relationships in which my MS is acknowledged are the healthiest, most nurturing relationships that I have. These are the spaces that I can be tired if I want, shaky if I happen to be shaky, or confused and losing words—and it is all okay. You know what else I have noticed? That when I have that space to be tired, shaky, and confused (and all other sorts of gimpy), that I am less tired, shaky, and confused than when I am trying to hide it or pretending that it doesn't really matter and that I am the same person that I have always been. Go figure.

There is no doubt that one of the worst aspects of MS can be, for many people, how it impacts them socially. All human relationships are complicated, but the intrusion of MS, with its often invisible and constantly shifting symptoms, can strain marriages, friendships, family interactions, and workplace dealings. Although many of these problems come from the other people, it is often we, the people with MS, who are contributing most to the awkwardness and strife by not feeling comfortable presenting our MS to the outside world.

Give MS an Appropriate Role in Your Relationships

Here's a newsflash: In case you hadn't noticed, MS can change dynamics in a relationship. These changes can exacerbate problems in relationships or they can make relationships stronger. They can be subtle differences, like a concerned glance from your spouse lingering an extra second when you are having trouble finding a word. They can be dramatic changes, like listening to your mom sniffle for the first 15 minutes of every conversation; being avoided by a friend who is uncomfortable that you have to use a cane sometimes or can't go outside in the summer; or, conversely, suddenly having an acquaintance blossom into a very good friend after she came to your rescue during a fatigue-filled day with an iced coffee and a shoulder to cry on.

Here is another secret that I will let you in on: People are complex, so complex that they often do not understand their own actions. This often results in them being unpredictable. In relationships, MS can make things feel "weird." In many circumstances this can be avoided and we can keep our relationships healthy. However, and this is a big, huge however, you cannot control other people's thoughts or actions, no matter what you do. It is up to us to do what we can to control ourselves and conduct ourselves in a dignified and loving manner in our dealings with others. That is what each of us can do—be the person that we would want to befriend.

Take Charge

Decide how you want to talk about MS in each of your relationships. Take control of the dialogue and deliberately create the relationship you want between your people and your MS.

All of us have different roles in the various relationships we are in, including those of daughter/son, spouse, parent, coworker, or friend. Just as each of these roles comes with unique modes of interaction and places in a hierarchy, our MS can affect each type of relationship differently. The uncertainty and changing abilities that come with this disease can lead to fear, resentment, stress, or loneliness in both the MSer and the other parties. Nevertheless, if handled strategically, the various relationships in your life can be protected from the negative impacts of MS to a great degree.

You (MSer) as Spouse/Partner

As trite as it may sound, MS can strengthen relationships as couples strategize how to work together as a team to compensate for the effects of MS. On the other hand, marriage and long-term relationships can be difficult for healthy people in the best of circumstances, and MS can certainly introduce impediments that change the whole vision of what both partners "signed up for." The person without MS may become the primary breadwinner or have to take on more parenting tasks.

The Real World

Never forget the "double whammy" our spouses deal with—less help from us and more MS-related tasks. We need to acknowledge them frequently.

The spouse or partner of a person with MS may also find that they are gradually (or suddenly) taking on a caregiving role. This may start out with little things, such as driving the MSer home after an MRI scan, but it can progress into providing more intimate kinds of help, like administering injections or assisting with hygiene needs. In this way, MS can transform a partnership between lovers to more of a parent-child situation, stripping people of dignity and introducing embarrassment and dependence, even though that is not intended.

The "collateral damage" from this shift in roles can be the death of a once-healthy sex life. Further alienation can occur when the person with MS begins to perceive themselves to be a burden, feels guilty, or stops talking to their partner about how they feel—in short, shutting the partner out emotionally while making more demands on him or her physically.

Make It Better

Make intimacy and sex a huge priority. You and your spouse need to figure this out.

At the risk of sounding trite (again), many of these problems can be avoided through good communication. Your partner needs to know how you are feeling, needs to know that his efforts are noticed—that all the work he is putting in is not going into a black hole. Your partner also needs to know that you are there for him, even if he needs to vent about your MS or discuss his own MS-related fears and emotions—in this case it is your job to listen. You both can take advantage of days, or even minutes, when the MS is less bad to enjoy your relationship through talking, laughing, and having sex.

The Real World

You can't blame MS for who you are or for who your spouse is. MS puts extra tension on relationships, but it doesn't change the fundamentals. You are still you and your spouse is still your spouse.

I am not unrealistic. If you are involved with a selfish pig, MS will surely not change that, and may speed up the demise of the relationship. Also, sometimes even good people cannot handle what MS has thrown at them through their partner, and a relationship that might be okay in wonderful circumstances will falter under this kind of stress.

The most important ingredients in a relationship are honesty, caring, and dignity. These will take you far, even far enough to be out of the long reach of MS.

You (MSer) as Parent

I was reduced to tears when one of my small daughters came to where I was sitting on the ground with my head in my hands, reeling from MS-related fatigue with a little vertigo thrown in, and adjusted my collar, saying, "Here you go, Mommy. I'll take care of you." I can tell you with certainty that young children pick up on the fact that something is wrong when a parent is not feeling well. This can manifest as increased clinginess, regression in terms of speech or potty training progress, or reversion to younger behavior (such as needing a pacifier). Children who are a little older may get worried that something terrible is happening—that their parent will die, that they will die, that they did something terrible and that whatever is going on is their fault. This may turn into sleeping issues or nightmares, withdrawing emotionally, or acting out at school.

Teenagers may be embarrassed about the whole situation, making them (even more) resentful and difficult to get along with. They may also go in the other direction, taking on emotional and physical responsibilities that put them in a caretaking or parent-type role.

The Real World

Don't forget that your children are entitled to their own reactions and emotions about your MS. While it is your MS, it is also your family's MS.

Before I had children, I was the most knowledgeable and most wonderful mother in the world—although I had no washcloths or diaper cream, I had brochures for cloth diapers and recipes for homemade organic baby food ready a couple months before they were born. You probably already guessed how far I got with those, so I will tell you this—we all have to make our own way as parents. I can't tell you what to do—I cannot tell you that you must be open about your MS with your children. I know that many people are uncomfortable with that, and I understand. The "experts" (most of whom do NOT have MS) say that we should answer all questions about our MS honestly and directly, adjusting the information as they get older. That might, or might not, work for you. I know that some people choose to keep the fact of their MS from their children until they reach a certain age or until something happens so that it must be revealed; they think that they are letting their children have a good shot at a normal life, without the pervasive worry of having a sick parent.

The only thing I can tell you with 100% clarity is that it is impossible to show your children too much love. As far as my situation goes, I have chosen to be very open with my daughters (in an age-appropriate way). I tell them when I am tired and I tell them when I feel better. They are still very small, but I intend to let them know about my MS as soon as it seems like they will understand. They have seen me give myself an injection, primarily out of practical necessity, as there was really nowhere and no time for me to have privacy at the moment. Honestly, I am kind of relieved that this is just part of who Mommy is to them and not a scary thing that I need to be secretive about.

We also need to remember that even when our children are grown and no longer live with us, we are still their parents, even if this relationship has come to closely resemble (or be) a friendship. We may require more help than before, but it is important to avoid leaning on our children too much emotionally or telling them intimate details of our lives better saved for our spouses, close friends, or therapists.

MSer as Child

My mom passed away about 6 months before I received my MS diagnosis, and I didn't even start experiencing the extreme symptoms that led to my diagnosis until after her death. As much as I miss her and would have loved to have been comforted by her, I also count my blessings that if she had to go so early, she did not have the extra pain of knowing about my MS. I knew her well—she would have obsessively worried about me and my future. I know myself well, too—this would have upset me greatly. I would have been sad for her worries and it would have heightened my own anxiety about the situation.

For those of you in the position of being a grown-up who faces the task of telling your parents that you have MS, I'll tell you something that may surprise you—this time, for a little while, your MS is not about you. If you are a parent, you know that you would much sooner take on any pain before allowing your child to experience just a fraction of the discomfort. It is no different for your parents, even though you are all grown up.

So, be gentle. Be understanding. Have your facts ready. Be calm. Try not to get upset when the tears come. Try to be patient when you hear the latest suggestion for a freaky remedy or hear something that Montel said repeated back to you for the tenth time. Your parents are trying to understand and help in their way. Don't shut them out, but do what you can to bring them to terms with your situation.

Of course, none of the above applies if you have a terrible relationship with one or both of your parents or if your MS is somehow used "against" you by them in any way.

MSer as Sibling, Close Friend, or Acquaintance

You know who the people in your life are and who you absolutely *need* to tell and for which reasons (she is your sister, he is your ex-husband who might need to take care of your child for a while if you have a relapse, she is your confidant to whom you tell everything). There are also people that definitely don't need to know anything about you (you fill in the blanks here).

Then there are a whole bunch of people who you might want to tell about your MS . . . or not. Take each person on a case-by-case basis. Some people you might want to tell because they went through health problems themselves and your gut tells you that they would be wonderful sources of support. Knowing about your MS might jointly benefit you and the other person in different ways— your child's teacher might be able to help him work through some worried or scared feelings he has about Mommy being so tired, or the neighbor could watch to make sure that your trash can gets to the curb in time for garbage collection. Then there are people who simply don't need to know, unless there is an extreme situation. You know who they are. Do not feel compelled to share all of your information with everyone, especially if it can be somehow used in a negative manner.

MSer as a Potential Romantic Interest

Dating is like going through puberty or being a brand-new mother—it can be terrifying (and terrible at times), but if you make it through okay, the rewards might be really good. If you are a person with MS who is in the early (or embryonic) stages of a relationship, you have two choices: (1) tell the other person about your MS, or (2) don't tell the other person about your MS. Of course, the loveliest outcome would be that you would tell the person, and they would say, "Oh, okay. That is no big deal, considering how fabulous, funny, and beautiful you are. What can I do to help?" Once we wake up from that fantasy (which, of course, could still happen), we worry about the following outcomes: (1) you tell the other person and it scares them away, or (2) you don't tell the other person and you are keeping a secret, which will either come out later or the relationship will perish before the truth is revealed.

I wish I could tell you what to do. You are pretty much on your own with this one, as we all have different personalities and find different types of partners interesting or desirable. What might have worked for me may not be a good idea for you. I will offer my opinion on one thing, however. We all pretty much know how a first date is going within about 15 minutes. Give it 30 minutes and we can guess with about 93% accuracy if we will see this person again. If you are thinking "probably not," there is really no need to say anything about the MS. If you are feeling the "vibe," I see no problem in mentioning it, despite the advice that you might get from "dating experts" (whoever those people are). I really think that if a person is going to be scared away, it will happen whether you tell them right away or after several dates. I also think if you wait longer than the aforementioned several dates to tell them, they may get nervous about a relationship because you were not honest from the beginning. On the other hand, your MS can be an excellent "loser screener," as another date following your MS disclosure indicates that this relationship may have excellent potential to become more serious.

Disclose Your MS with Class (And Compassion)

Now that I have been officially diagnosed with MS for a number of years, pretty much all of my friends and family members and most of my slightly-better-than-casual acquaintances know that I have it. I am not a person who is that private about medical things—in fact, my people probably wish I was a little more quiet about some of the health-related things that I share (I am certain that this was the case during my twin pregnancy). However, after I was first diagnosed and the time came to tell different people about my new status as a person with MS, I can tell you that I made many mistakes in how I let people know about my diagnosis.

I guess I kind of forgot that most of these people had not been traveling the emotional road to diagnosis with me. I just kind of "put it all out there" in a very blunt, and what I thought was a matter-of-fact, way. The reactions ranged from tears to shocked silence to "I guess it could be worse" sort of comments, all of which kind of surprised me. In retrospect, I believe that it was more my lame delivery than it was the person's response that made the situation awkward.

Take Charge

Know what your goal is when you talk about your MS. Are you looking for sympathy? For support? Do you just want to shock someone? Make sure your communication and goals are linked to each other.

Here are some tips to make disclosing your MS status more palatable to you and the person you are telling:

Avoid shocking people (unless you want to). Set up this part of the conversation a little. Start by saying something like, "I have some news to tell you that isn't so great," or "There is something that I would like to share with you because you are my friend." Though this may seem a little staged, it is better than, "Hi, yeah, just wanted to let you know that I was just diagnosed with multiple sclerosis. And, no, that does not make me one of Jerry's Kids. Anyway, gotta go."

Use details. Part of reducing the shock factor is the use of relevant details. If you simply tell someone that you have MS, they are left to fill in these details themselves, and (trust me) the first things that come to mind are sad and scary images from news stories of people who died from MS or a friend's uncle who was bedridden. If you tell your story—including your freaky symptoms, your suspicions that something was wrong, and the funny or creepy doctors that you encountered—you give the other person something to relate to. They can get involved with the narrative and picture you going through these things. The MS then becomes part of the story, not a shocking bomb that is dropped.

Tell with feeling. I think what freaked many people out in my delivery was my kind of numb and somber delivery. Be sure to use a lot of energy—positive and/or negative—in your story. This will allow your listener to see how the MS is affecting you and how to gauge their own reaction.

Make your listeners characters in your story. Maybe they helped you a few times when you were fatigued. Maybe you yelled at them when feeling stressed. Maybe you want to ask them for help in the event of a relapse or worsening of symptoms. Including them in the story will not only hold their interest, but it will also open up the possibility of them being part of your story in the future. This will also make the story into a dialogue and allow them to ask questions of their own.

Use These Communication "Cheat Sheets"

It's a terrible situation, and one that I have found myself in far too often. You feel awful and want to communicate that to a loved one, but you feel too awful to find the right words, so you use the wrong words. A fight or misunderstanding occurs, which makes you feel more awful for all new and different reasons.

I have thought about this for a long time. As a writer, I treasure words. I delight in the English language. We have words to explain every nuance, every shade of gray, with incredible precision and artistry. That is, until you are really desperate to get your point across because you are under physical and emotional duress caused by one MS symptom or another—at the time that you need to explain things accurately and concisely, in a way that people will understand and react with empathy, your words seem to abandon you. I am always telling my toddler twins to "use their words," yet I can easily find myself later flapping my hands around when trying to explain a complex emotion to my husband or a friend, with the only words at my disposal being "Fix it." or "Go. A. Way. Now."

I find myself lying awake at night and replaying many conversations, using the words I wish I could have found at the moment that I needed them. I decided to do us all a favor and put down some of these thoughts for us to use at critical moments. Feel free to read from the book, to point to the paragraphs, to write these ideas out in your own words, adapting them to make them just right. If you feel strange about using the words of a stranger to "talk" to your loved ones, think about the greeting card aisle on Valentine's Day and all those big, slightly befuddled men reading dozens of cards until they find just the right one to communicate "I love you" to someone they see every day. Hallmark knows that we all need a little help sometimes—they just haven't gotten around to making the MS greeting card line yet, so I went ahead and did it for them (with fewer rhymes and no smiling puppy or laughing kitten illustrations).

"I am tired."

Saying the words "I am tired" isn't really accurate. That is because the right words to describe exactly how I feel don't seem to exist. I could use all the metaphors or comparisons to something you might have felt in the past (jet lag with a hangover, a heavy wet blanket over my head), but really, they fall short. Attempts to put words to it might come across to you as overly dramatic, exaggerated, or maudlin—and knowing you thought that I was any of those things would only make me feel worse.

Let's keep it at this: When I feel this way, my limitations define me in many ways. I am unable to think clearly, I am dizzy, I am nauseated. I cannot fake my way through this unique type of exhaustion. I am depleted, and these are the times that I have to admit, even to myself, that I am not entirely whole or healthy.

I am telling you this because I want you to know about this aspect of multiple sclerosis, which, unfortunately is also a part of me. This will not last forever. I will have times, hopefully soon, when I feel intact again. I will be more functional. Until then, I need acceptance. I know that this is also frustrating and scary to you, and you are not forgotten.

Do Your Best

Practice your communication. There may be big difference between what you think you said, what you actually said, and how someone understood what you said. Words like "tired" or "bad day" may have very different meanings when spoken by someone with MS. Be sure to communicate what you mean.

"I am sad/angry."

I know all of it—I know that there are people that have it worse than me. I know that being angry or sad doesn't help me get better. I know that it's not considered healthy to wallow in negative feelings.

I also know that I don't really care about all of that right now (and maybe don't even believe it all). Multiple sclerosis has stolen something, many things, from me. I am angry and sad about the things I have lost (feeling good, thinking clearly, being able to plan from day to day, being "normal") and the things that I have gained (physical pain, worry about getting worse, confusion, daily reminders that I am living with a chronic and unpredictable disease).

I am not blaming anyone for these feeling, although that would be easier. I am sorry if I lash out at you or turn away from you. I need to battle with these things right now. I will come back. I need patience more than anything, and a little space to finish this round of the fight.

I also know that you may be sad and angry, too. Let's both try to remember that it's the MS, and not us, that is the cause of these feelings.

"I just can't right now."

I want to, I really do. I would love to [fill in the blank] more than you know. I know it would be good for me to leave the house/be with people/have fun. I want to be like a "normal" person and make plans and keep them. I want little outings to be fun and not fill me with dread, wondering how bad I will feel and spending time strategizing how to make it through the situation or get out of it gracefully. I want to be the person who grabs her sweater or binoculars or sunglasses and says, "Come on! Let's go! What are you waiting for?" as I beat you out the door.

But I just can't right now. I'm sorry. Maybe next time. Ask me again, please.

"I need help."

This is not easy for me to say, but I need help. Because of my MS [elaborate here if necessary], I am unable to [fill in the blank] without assistance. Will you help me get this done?

"I love you."*

I love you.

* I cannot count the number of times that I attempted to write (then erased) this particular little helper script for us all. I finally came to the realization that these simple words will do the trick if they are said in a heartfelt way, and that adding in additional verbiage about MS or pain or being sorry that you have MS just messes up the whole thing somehow. It helps to be holding the person's hand and looking directly into his or her eyes when you say it. You can also pick up the phone and achieve pretty much the same effect, as long as there is no TV on, children competing for attention, or dinner that needs constant stirring on the stove—just you and the other person connecting for long enough to tell them these words.

By the way, I recommend the same technique for saying "Thank you."

A Special Note—"Help Now!!!"

For all the advice and scripts and pushes to "just communicate what you need," there will be moments that you urgently require help, only to find that your power of communication has completely left you. I have had moments when I am too hot, too fatigued, too scared, and/or too confused to let my husband know that I need him to come home immediately, or help me out of the car, or do anything else. I have ended up trying to explain things in a rambling sort of way that just served to frighten and frustrate him, when all I really needed was to clutch his elbow to get from one place to another until I could pull myself together. I recommend that you discuss this situation with your spouse, close friend, or loved ones, and come up with a code word that means "Help now!!!" Think of something that does not sound too alarming to other people, but rather just lets the other person know that they are needed. For instance, I might forgo using "Code red!" or "Situation critical!" in lieu of a cute little secret code phrase, such as "A lime daiquiri sounds lovely right now," or something about a favorite Dr. Seuss character. Remember, the goal is to get the help you need right away without making anyone too flustered. The discussion about why you need help and your emotions about the situation can come later.

Get Help

I know that the more urgently that I need help, the more flustered and inarticulate I become, which makes me panic more. My husband and I have worked out a code, so that whenever I mention that I really "need new shoes," he calmly, but quickly, comes to my aid without alarming our daughters or alerting anyone else that I am freaking out.

Assess People

We all have people in our lives. Some of these people are helpful and some are not. Some understand what it is like to have a chronic illness like MS, some do not. Some people make us feel better, and others make us feel worse. We often don't realize the impact people have on us or our MS until things blow up or we have spent too much time feeling bad about ourselves, not realizing that maybe we don't need certain people in our lives. Conversely, we may take supportive people for granted, just because they have always been there for us, and we neglect to give them the attention that they deserve. At some point it is good to take a close, objective-as-possible look at the people in our lives and decide if we need to change our relationships in some way.

> ### Take Charge
>
> Try to make the most helpful people the ones that you deal with regularly. Don't leave any social support that is available to you untapped.

By answering a few targeted questions about the people in your life, you'll create an opportunity to discover how these relationships impact your MS. This will help you determine what actions to take in order to construct a social environment that increases your health. Without taking the time to think about how the people around you affect your MS, you may be creating or perpetuating negative situations or missing opportunities for support.

Here are your steps to assessing people:

Make a list. Make a list of the important people in your life. List everyone, even people that you have a connection with but do not see regularly. Also, be sure to list people that you see once a week or more (coworkers, people from church, people in a club). Include all the people you talk with on the phone, communicate with by e-mail, or chat with online.

Score them. For each person, decide how supportive that person would be in a crisis, on a scale of 1 to 10. You would give a 1 to a person who makes things worse, and a 10 to a person who is completely and utterly helpful and supportive, with most people falling somewhere in the middle. Place the person's score to the left of his or her name. You can leave a blank next to anyone you feel like you don't know well enough, but try to make a guess about how they would respond if you called on them for help.

Score them again. Next, give each of the people a score, on a scale of 1 to 10, based on how much you talk to these people about your MS or other problems. Write this number to the right of the name. People you talk to the most about your MS and other problems get a 10, and people to whom you've never mentioned your MS or other problems get a 1, with most people receiving scores between these two extremes.

Assess your people. Look over your list. Do the people with a 10 on the left also have a 10 on the right? Are the people who are most supportive the ones you talk with about your MS? If the lists don't look the same, you may have a great deal of untapped support.

Make a plan. For each of the people who scored high on the "support-ive" list (the one to the left of the name), write out one thing they can do to help you right now or in the future. Maybe they would be good at figuring out a symptom. Maybe they could help relieve your stress. Maybe you could spend an afternoon with them just having fun. Maybe they are good at searching the Internet for information. Maybe they would just be good at listening to you. For each person, find one thing they could do to help.

You need to be able to rely on people and know they will be there for you. You might ask someone just to respond to a question by e-mail, to tell her story about how she coped with something difficult in her own life, or to help you more directly. Look over your list or come up with something new. For a little challenge, ask at least three different people to do one thing this week. Practice asking for help.

Tips for Increasing Social Support

You don't have to directly ask people for help—some people do it natu-rally. Just pick up the phone and talk with someone about what is on your mind. That counts.

Many people say they are afraid to be a burden, but often what is behind that is the fear of exposing oneself. MS can be scary, but if you keep all of your emotions about it bottled up inside, you can blow the scariness out of proportion. Instead talk with people who are support-ive. They can help keep your thoughts and feelings about your MS in perspective.

Get Help

No one can help if you don't ask. Be considerate, specific, and respectful when you ask for help and people will gladly pitch in.

Don't overlook people. You may be surprised how helpful an occasional acquaintance, a coworker, or a friend from church can be. By talking about your MS and asking for help, you are reaching out and making a connection. If you just keep answering "Fine" in response to the question "How are you?" you are shutting people out.

Don't just complain to people. It's not about getting sympathy—it's about getting help with the things you need. Be sure to figure out how to return the help and make the relationship mutual.

Make an effort to increase your social support. Take time this week to reconnect with old friends, to get out more and to meet new people. Spend time thinking about ways you can increase the number of people you come into contact with. Find organizations to join and people to spend time with. Don't do things alone, call and invite people to come with you. Spend some real effort here—you never know whom you might meet or when a so-so friendship might mature into something wonderful.

Take Care of Your Caregivers

I am grateful to my neurologist for many things, but one thing that will always stand out in my mind is a moment during my initial consult with him. He had shown me pretty big areas of brain atrophy in my MRI, he said that I probably had been living with MS for 15 or 20 years, and he told me that he wasn't sure if some of the symptoms I was experiencing would ever go away. After that litany, I was understandably surprised when he then told me that I was very lucky. "You have him," he said, pointing to my husband. "That's better than anything I will ever be able to do for you."

With those words, he not only put things in perspective for me in terms of how truly fortunate I am to have such a relationship, but he also (perhaps unintentionally) placed a pretty heavy burden on my husband's shoulders. I was beginning my journey with MS, and it suddenly became our adventure in a very real way. I am pretty reluctant to throw the word "caregiver" around, as it conjures up images of people who are caring for people who are bedridden or have frank dementia and require full-time care to get basic needs met. However, the people closest to us *are* often taking care of us to varying degrees.

The Real World

It may be a little difficult to get your head around the word "caregiver" in relation to your situation. It was for me. Use a different word (or no word at all), but do not fail to recognize and acknowledge those things that certain people do for us.

Most of us fall somewhere closer to the middle of the spectrum. You may be in a situation in which you do need help to do most things. More likely, though, you can do many things for yourself, but need a little extra help and understanding to accomplish some of the things you used to do or would like to do. It might be seemingly easy and effortless things like an extra reminder to take your medications or help chopping vegetables for dinner. It may be a little more involved, in that you need to be driven to most places. Of course, some of us do require more intimate care, such as help bathing or using the restroom. Although it is easy to think that these things are "no big deal," especially for those of us who just need a helping hand occasionally, think back to our pre-MS days. Often a niggling little request from someone or an errand that I had to do was enough to throw me off my whole tightly-choreographed routine and send me into a tailspin.

So, how do we ensure that those people that help us stay energetic and happy?

Acknowledge their contribution (and burden). My husband mentioned to me the other day that when I am doing poorly, everyone asks about me, but no one ever asks him how he is doing. He gets less attention than usual, even though he is also dealing with increased responsibilities and stress. He is right. It is important to remember that these people are not only taking on extra things for us, but that they also lost much of our contribution to the "team."

It is crucial that we make an effort to recognize and remind our caregivers (or whatever you want to call them) of everything that they do and how much MS has affected their lives, too. Many people in the "helper role" feel strange or guilty thinking of themselves as "burdened," because they compare themselves to us, the people with MS, and think about our losses, symptoms, and problems. This makes it difficult to face the fact that they need help or support. Remember, these people in our lives are both taking on the things we cannot do, as well as taking on extra tasks that come along with helping us.

Keep them informed. Studies have shown that people in caregiving roles benefit from having as much knowledge as possible about the disease. It is much easier for people to deal with something if they understand something about the "enemy," especially since they do not have the direct physical experience of MS symptoms. It is important that at least the basic information about the disease comes from other sources besides you—however, you should also share information about specific symptoms that you are having with your caregiver. Show them articles that describe what you are feeling or what you are worried about.

Encourage them to find support. Some caregiver resources include:

National Family Caregivers Association (www.thefamilycaregiver.org) works to educate, support, and speak up for the more than 50 million Americans who care for loved ones. Their mission is "to empower family caregivers to act on behalf of themselves and their loved ones, and to remove barriers to health and well being." They do this by linking caregivers to one another in different ways and teaching them to advocate for themselves through a volunteer program called Caregiver Community Action Network (CCAN) and through a small online forum. They also have a comprehensive curriculum called "Communicating Effectively with Healthcare Professionals," which is comprised of video classes and a series of downloadable forms and articles. They publish a quarterly print and online newsletter called *TAKE CARE!— Self Care for the Family Caregiver.* They can be found online or reached at 800-896-3650.

Well Spouse Association (www.wellspouse.org) is an organization that primarily assists people who are caring for a disabled spouse. Services include informing spouses about a national network of support groups; facilitating a mentor program and round robin letter writing groups; organizing regional respite weekends and a national conference for caregivers; and providing continuing support for members whose spouses have died. Well Spouse Association also publishes a newsletter, called *Mainstay,* and an e-newsletter. The Well Spouse Web site contains information about coping and survival skills and includes an online forum for spousal caregivers. The Well Spouse Association can be reached by phone at 800-838-0879.

Today's Caregiver (www.caregiver.com) offers a print and an online version of the *Today's Caregiver* magazine. It also runs a small forum and an online store with books and videos.

Diversify your team. Even if the majority of extra responsibility will fall to one person, it is much less overwhelming for everyone if there is a backup plan. I know that on the days that my husband was out of town and the care of my infant twins fell entirely to me, I felt tired before I even got around to feeding the second baby her breakfast. But when I realized that my aunt was just a phone call away, the same amount of work was much easier. Ask other people for help, or at least to be on call, in addition your spouse or the person who always helps you. I remember once hearing that "If you want someone to be your friend, ask them for help." Many people love to be asked for assistance and would love to do something for you, but they need you to make a specific request.

Also, there are many services that are free of charge or very low cost that can lessen the load in terms of tasks or errands that might fall to other people. I love to cook, but often have a hard time getting to the store. In the past, I would feel bad about asking my husband to track down funky ingredients or do a "big shop." This would result in picking up take-out food that we didn't really like or surviving on sandwiches. I then discovered that our local grocery store had a "personal shopper" service that was free of charge. I now e-mail them my list, with all sorts of obscure ingredients on it, and *voila!*—later that afternoon, my husband calls from the parking lot and sits in the car while the bags are placed in the trunk.

Make It Better

Do everything in your power to make your caretakers' jobs easier. Give easy-to-follow instructions, find ways to save time, and tell them to take some time off when you are having a good day.

Be a team. Again, keep in mind that our helpers not only have the stress of doing extra stuff, they also have a front-row seat to the spectacle of our increasing (temporary or permanent) disability. It is essential that living with this disease be a team effort. Yes, we are the people with MS, but it is often the disease and not us that is setting the bar and making the decisions for us. My husband puts it well when he says, "I know that you want to go out, but I am asking the MS if it is a good idea." Putting it this way alleviates my guilt (at least somewhat) when I have to say no to plans. It is the MS messing things up again, so we find something else to do together.

Take care of the caregiver. Everyone needs time off. Encourage your helpers to take breaks and do something they enjoy, even if it means that you can't come along.

Constantly improve and experiment. Always be thinking of better ways to do things, from modifications of your bathroom and kitchen to consolidating your grocery list so that you can do all the weekly shopping in one trip. Any improvement in efficiency helps both you and your caregiver.

Bringing Your MS to Work (or Not)

This is not a section about working with MS, whether you should keep working, or what your rights are—these topics are touched upon in the section entitled "Workplace independence" in Chapter 7. The following discussion is about acknowledging and figuring out what we want from the relationships that come along with being in the workplace.

There are many kinds of relationships in the workplace. You have your superiors, your coworkers, the people who work for you, and perhaps a whole bunch of other people that keep the place running in some way but have nothing to do with you directly. Your relationships with these various people might be friendly, adversarial, collaborative, or competitive.

Take Charge

Your human resources department may be a confidential place to see about some accommodations at work. The HR people should be able to make things happen without having to tell your manager or coworkers the reason.

It's kind of a weird situation, when you think about it. People working full-time often spend more time with the people at their workplace than they do with their spouses or children—certainly this is the case during the week. For many valid reasons, often people with MS do not disclose their status to these people that they see every Monday through Friday. However, not mentioning your MS doesn't make it go away—in fact, people who choose not to tell anyone are faced with the additional stress of hiding symptoms, compensating for fatigue and diminishing abilities, and living with a big secret. On the other hand, once you disclose, people are watching you more closely to see how the MS is affecting you, including your work. It's a conundrum, no doubt, one that must be worked out by each individual after a number of factors are considered.

Here are some questions to ask yourself as you think about telling people in the workplace about your MS:

Why do I want to disclose my MS? Just take the time to think about the answer to this question. Maybe you just are tired of having a secret. Maybe you are feeling that specific symptoms are interfering with your work and you want to explain this to people.

How do I want to disclose my MS? If you are presenting your MS as a problem, consider how you could also offer a solution. Maybe there are some accommodations that might help you do your job better that you would like to suggest to your boss as options. Really think about this. Things like changing your schedule around to avoid being in the office during peak fatigue hours or working from home some days might make a huge difference. You may need the temperature turned down a little in your area (in the case of heat intolerance) or to be moved to a quieter place to work (if you have cognitive dysfunction).

If you are telling coworkers about your MS, think about what it will mean to them if you are able to take on less work some days. Consider things from their point of view, then think about what you would want to hear if you were in their place. In many cases, it would be really helpful to prepare people to do stuff that they usually rely on you for with the least amount of effort (see the section on "Prepare for a relapse or symptom worsening" in Chapter 7 for more detailed information on this). Give them the tools they need to work effectively in your absence.

What is the best/worst/most probable result of disclosing my MS? We all hope for certain responses when we tell people we have MS. In the workplace, it seems like an ideal response would be something along the lines of, "You are so brave for telling us and your exemplary work would never have offered any clue that you had any problems. Of course, we want to do anything to keep you healthy and happy, so please let us know of any accommodations that we can make for you to ensure that you are able to stay with us. Effective immediately, we are cutting your workload by half and giving you a bonus, just for being so wonderful." You can indulge in a similar little fantasy for a while, but it is important to really think through all the scenarios that you can imagine. That way, you can respond rationally (rather than emotionally) to anything that happens, which increases your odds for the best possible outcome.

Things to Consider Before Disclosing at Work:

Again, before you disclose your MS status, think through the situation. As someone who has a tendency to blurt things out then wonder what the heck just happened, I will tell you that there are some truisms in life, some of which are not pretty, which will apply to your workplace situation:

Information spreads. It just does. You know it as well as I do, people cannot keep secrets. Think about all the "intel" that you have helped travel around the office, whether it was in a gossipy or a matter-of-fact manner. Trust me, your disclosure will not have immunity from this network. Keep this in mind when you tell your office buddy about your MS, your urinary incontinence, your cognitive dysfunction, or your occasional use of medical marijuana.

In most situations, a person's first (or second) thought is "How will this affect me?" Even the nicest person will get here eventually. In a workplace, even friendly relationships often have an element of professional give-and-take or teamwork that may be affected by your inability to perform like you used to.

People usually want to do the right thing. They do. You can help them to know what the right thing is by straight out telling them, "You know what would really help me is if you . . ." If you make people feel like they are part of a "team," they will want to pitch in. Start with things like asking them to condense their 27 daily e-mail messages into one document or run interference with a particularly tiring client. Make sure you thank them for their help.

What about disclosing during an interview? The National Multiple Sclerosis Society recommends NOT disclosing MS status in a job interview, suggesting that you focus instead on the job in question and your abilities to perform the necessary work, even if you will eventually need accommodations. Prospective employers are legally not permitted to ask why you need a mobility device.

While I am pretty sure that omitting your MS status from a discussion of your abilities is very sound advice from the NMSS, it's kind of hard for me to imagine leaving the fact of my MS out of a request to "tell me a little about yourself." This is something that you may have to discuss with a couple of friends and loved ones to figure out your approach to in different situations.

The Bottom Line

It's kind of fascinating to watch toddlers get increasingly frustrated when they cannot get people to completely bend to their will. People will say, "It's time for them to learn that they don't control the universe. After all, they are already three." I agree, until I realize that it took me about 40 years to understand that, no matter how hard I try, I cannot control how people are going to behave in a relationship. People that you love might betray you, and people that don't even show up on your radar often may come to your rescue.

The Real World

You can't control how people will react to your MS, but you can control how and what you tell them. Be thoughtful and goal-driven when talking about your MS.

It also has recently dawned on me that you can really only expect people to be who they are. I have wasted countless hours of stress, sadness, and anger over the actions or lack of action of people who were not filling in all the gaps that I needed filled in a friendship. It has truly been liberating to finally realize that some people would always be late, some people would not be able to grapple with complex emotional issues, and some people were focused on completely different things than those that I found important. Once this finally sunk in,

I was able to have much healthier, happier relationships with people whose friendship I truly cherished, as I enjoyed and valued those people for who they were, instead of agonizing over who they weren't.

All this is to say that we can only control ourselves. The bitch of it all is, as people with MS, we can't even do that all the way. The MS may cause us to be so tired that we have to cancel plans, it may make us forget important dates or conversations, and it may make us needier than we would like to be. The best we can do is to be people who we can be proud of, regardless of the circumstances.

10

Cooperate with Your Emotions

I wish I had some pithy story to write here that would make it obvious to everyone that I have transcended any negative emotions about having MS. I would love to be so Zen-like about the whole thing that readers would feel my words glowing, radiating love and acceptance, indicating that I have truly reached Nirvana and I am at peace with my MS and see the destruction that is being unleashed in my central nervous system as part of a bigger, universal plan. Well, the words aren't glowing, because that isn't the case.

I'm far from serene about this whole friggin' mess. I'm angry and I'm hateful at times. I lash out at my most beloved people in the world at the very times that I am feeling lonely and scared and in need of love. I withdraw, I cry, and I feel sorry for myself. I lie to myself about all the fabulous physical feats that I could have performed and career paths that would have led me to greatness, if only it wasn't for MS messing it all up.

Then, much like I feel after watching the news or certain reality shows, I just get tired of myself and that whole storyline. I need some relief from the angry person inside that I cannot get away from. I need to find something about myself to be proud of, before my hatred of this disease becomes difficult to separate from my measure of self-worth. I find a way to look outside of myself—I pray, I cook, I read, I play a made-up version of Candyland with my daughters.

It's inescapable, living with this disease and making choices about how to proceed in your life with MS is fraught with feelings. As you try to look at statistics and likelihoods when making decisions about treatments or future plans, your emotions may pull you away from looking at things scientifically and acting rationally. You will learn that not only is it okay to act in accord with emotions, it is desirable to give your feelings "a vote" in important matters, or underlying worry and stress will always be present. It is also crucial to understand when negative feelings become destructive and need to be addressed (and how to do it).

Tune In to Your Instincts

Every so often, a thought will enter my head that is completely unrelated to what I am doing at the moment, and I will try to squash it and make it go away because I fear that it is not just a random "isn't that strange" type of thing, but a premonition of something—which is pretty much always unpleasant.

For example, I'm standing at the kitchen sink washing dishes and thinking about the next exciting thing in my daily repertoire, when out of nowhere, I will think, "Hmm. It's been a couple of months since one of the girls has been sick. Seems like we are due for something." Weird. I wonder what made me think that just then. I stop what I am doing and go have a look at them. Clearly I am just being silly, as they are alternating squealing with delight with negotiations of who gets to be Simba the lion and who has to be a hyena in their game (with little breaks of racing around the furniture). They have never looked healthier or more active.

Fast forward three hours. I'm holding a twin who has just vomited on me wondering what to do about the other one who has slipped in the vomit, fallen backwards and hit her head.

Though I would love to believe that I am psychic and have powers that I could then use to gain all sorts of fame and riches, I don't really think that is it. My theory is that something in my primal brain instinctively sensed that something was amiss long before the vomiting incident happened. Maybe my daughter's eyes weren't quite as bright as usual, maybe there was a smell that was undetectable, but that made it to some prehistoric, maternal neurological center that flagged it as "not right." Of course, I then overrode that by gathering empirical evidence that reassured me that my gut was wrong.

We all have experiences when we just know something *just isn't right*. In my example above, there really wasn't anything I could have done to stop the chain of events. However, many of us have these feelings of vague unease or flashes of "don't do it" when we are faced with a decision. Conversely, we also might just have a feeling that something is right, that it is good, that this is the path we should take—many happily married people say that about their spouse as they recall the first time they laid eyes on the person.

In his book, *Blink: The Power of Thinking Without Thinking*, Malcolm Gladwell refers to a phenomenon similar to this as "thin-slicing"—the "ability of our unconscious to find patterns in situations and behaviors based on very narrow slices of experience."[1] The theory behind thin-slicing is that our unconscious is conducting an accelerated analysis of a combination of experience, knowledge, emotion, and instincts to give us a flash answer of "right" or "wrong," "good" or "bad."

Do Your Best

Some questions have no right answer and no amount of research will get you there. Whether you are choosing a symptom management approach or deciding whether to tell a coworker about your MS, remember to do a "gut check," too.

Turn to any given page in this book and I have probably written words there pleading with each of you to do your homework, gather your information, monitor this and assess that aspect of your life, including your friends, your MS, your doctor, and your future plans. I am going to take a teeny-tiny break from that to tell you that in order to live a life filled with conviction and forward inertia, you must learn to trust your gut. Not only that, you must have the confidence to be able to act on what your instincts are telling you.

This will apply to different situations as you live your life with MS.

You may have a symptom that doesn't really seem that dramatic to an observer, but that you know signals a relapse—which gets confirmed by an MRI. You may have a very uneasy feeling about a treatment plan, but go along with your family and doctor as they "strongly encourage" you to take it, only to spend a couple of months lying awake at night regretting your decision, as you focus on potential side effects and freak out every time you hear a report of an adverse event connected to this medication. You may have a good relationship with someone at work, so despite some hesitation and a little anxiety, you disclose your MS status and that you feel like you are "slipping" a little cognitively, only to find out a week later that she has told everyone in the office, and that your clients are now being given to someone else.

Although your instincts might not have gone to medical school or have an MRI image of your brain to refer to, your gut feelings are often a vital component in making important decisions and bringing up questions to help you find your comfort level. Don't get me wrong: I am still a fan of researching a subject (to death), but one component of your exploration or investigation should be checking in with how your gut perceives the situation, which most people try to squash by piling more statistics and papers onto the feelings. Here are some questions to help bring your gut instinct into the equation when making a decision:

- What was my *very first feeling* when I felt that symptom, heard that recommendation, talked to that person?
- Have I had this feeling about something before? Was I right?
- If I am considering something that still leaves me with a feeling of unease, why am I doing it? Are friends, family, or my doctor pushing me to do this? Did I do some research that gave me information that lead to this decision? Am I taking the easier path than the one my gut is telling me to take?
- Will taking the path that I have chosen lead to additional stress, worry, or questioning?

Honor Your Feelings, But Stop When You Are Done

When I have a question or am approaching a topic that feels bigger than me, I typically go to the scientists to see what they have discovered. Doing a search in PubMed, however, involving the emotions of people with MS actually intensified my feelings of anger, fear, anxiety, sadness, self-pity, and loneliness connected with my disease. The researchers are trying to figure out how these emotions impact us physically and mentally by deconstructing what we do with them, whether it is drink excessively, be non-adherent to prescribed treatment regimens, burn out our caregivers, or spiral into depression. Of course, the scientists also want to help us cope with our potentially "destructive" feelings and have done some more research to come up with a variety of solutions, including: giving people comprehensive information when they are diagnosed, encouraging us to exercise, recommending that nurses ask about our emotional well-being, and suggesting a course of psychotherapy. I don't know—to me, much of it seems a little simplistic and not quite applicable to the realities of trying to cope, and thrive, while living with MS. I guess this is because emotions are complex and personal and always seem pretty distilled (and even misinterpreted) by people without MS, including researchers.

Take Charge

Be angry, be sad, be afraid, be lonely—then stop. Repeat when necessary. Just don't forget to stop.

So, as a person actually living with MS, I'll offer up an account of what these emotions feel like to me. I am sure that your experience with all of them is different, but equally valid. In my opinion, "speaking the truth" about these often-ugly feelings helps them do their good work of helping us process undesirable things that are often beyond our control, but it also helps limit their potential for destruction.

Anger. I'll go first—I get angry, really angry. And when I am told or I read somewhere that I need to "get over" or "work through" my anger in order to be healthy and deal effectively with my MS, that makes me angrier. You probably have your own reasons for being angry at and about your MS. Some of these might be global, as in "I am angry that I cannot continue to work full-time" or "I am angry that I have to inject myself." Others might be around very specific symptoms or situations—"I am angry that I can't go to the birthday party for my friend's daughter because it is outside during the hottest part of the day" or "I am angry that I couldn't keep up with the conversation at dinner with my friends last night."

The Real World

Your anger is waiting, looking for an excuse to come out. Don't confuse the excuse with the real source, in many cases, your MS.

Though it is hard to control sometimes, realize that anger is often expressed as irritability or sarcasm directed at those that happen to just be standing in the way of it. Try not to lash out at those innocent bystanders. It can also come out at unexpected times in a completely overblown reaction to something small. In her insightful and articulate book, *Life Disrupted: Getting Real About Chronic Illness in Your Twenties and Thirties,* Laurie Edwards recounts an incident in which she had a self-described "meltdown" over the wrong salad dressing being included with a delivery order dinner. She talks about weeping inconsolably after flinging the salad in the trashcan, and finding it difficult to articulate why the "crappy Greek dressing symbolized all the tiny little aggravations that had accumulated over the years."[2]

Fear and anxiety. Right after I was diagnosed, fear and anxiety were my predominant emotions. In my case, many things that I was afraid of in the beginning have come to pass—I have had to learn how to inject myself, I have had many of the different symptoms that I dreaded at one time or another, I have had to stop driving, I have become incredibly heat intolerant, and testing has confirmed my worries that I have lost some of my IQ points to cognitive dysfunction. By necessity, however, I have incorporated many of these former "things to be feared" into my life, and it has occurred to me that the things that seemed the scariest at the beginning turned out not to be so terrifying when they were actually happening.

Don't Panic

MS is scary; it is. Make it less scary by turning unknowns into knowns and uncontrollables into controllables whenever you can.

Much fear comes from uncertainty, from being unable to control the future. When you are in the midst of being afraid, it doesn't help to recognize the fact that, for most people, MSers or not, "control" is an illusion anyway. Any of us could have our lives turned upside down by financial losses, natural disasters, or one of our family members being diagnosed with a health problem. Clearly, those of us with MS and our family members do live with a specific kind of uncertainty and must be able to respond—rather than freezing up—making it necessary to find the balance between living in abject fear of disease progression and ignoring real changes that need attention.

If fear or anxiety stemming from uncertainty lasts for too long, people may do harmful and impulsive things to try to gain control. They may begin to alter their treatment plan without telling their doctor and turn to potentially dangerous complementary and alternative medicine approaches. They may also make drastic changes to their lives, such as moving, leaving relationships or solidifying unhealthy ones, or quitting jobs. Although it is very difficult to do while in the grasp of fear, it is crucial to distinguish between things that can be controlled and those that cannot. We can then strategize how to manage the things that we can influence and adapt to the things beyond our immediate control.

Sadness. Sadness is a tough one. Anger and anxiety are "volatile" and can often be lessened after an outburst or change of scenery. Sadness, on the other hand, is just "heavy." Researchers say that sadness in MS can be traced to self-pity that may come from lost abilities, the perceived loss of abilities, or the connected realization that some things that you might have imagined yourself doing that are no longer possible (given physical limitations or other obstacles) have arisen because of MS. Prolonged sadness can become "chronic sorrow," which is linked to certain losses felt by people with MS: loss of hope, loss of control over the body, loss of a healthy identity, loss of integrity and dignity, loss of faith that life is fair, loss of relationships, and loss of freedom.[3] It is precisely these losses that we must strive to counter in our quest for quality of life.

A special note about sadness: if you have MS and feel very sad or have no interest in things around you, you need to seek help—especially if you have had these feelings for two weeks or more and they are interfering with your daily life. Depression is a very common symptom of multiple sclerosis. It is nothing to be embarrassed about, it is not your fault and it can be treated.

Loneliness. You are right: *they* don't understand. However, you don't really need them to. Invisible symptoms are very difficult for others to comprehend, and much of my loneliness comes from people actually trying to connect by relating discomforts or problems that they have to my MS symptoms—"I get tired, too." or "I haven't been able to remember anything either since I had kids." Maybe even worse is when people try to make me feel better in a patronizing way—"You're doing great for someone with MS. If you feel as bad as you say, it's amazing that you get anything done." I'd rather be accused of being lazy or ditzy than have someone feel like they have to encourage me.

Make It Better

Talk to people who *do* understand you and the full range of your emotions about having MS. Make an effort to cultivate friends who are also living with the disease.

We often avoid contact with others when we are feeling our worst, most affected by our symptoms, having the hardest time emotionally, being afraid to burden people or be pitied. This, however, is precisely when we need contact the most.

Honor Your Negative Emotions

How can we interact with these emotions in a way that we get what we need from them, but still are able to escape? In my opinion, it is a good thing to occasionally wallow in these emotions. Trevis Gleason, in his blog for Everyday Health, "Life with MS" (www.everydayhealth.com/blog/trevis-life-with-multiple-sclerosis-ms), expresses it the following way:

> "I look at anger (and this also works for pity, sadness and depression, etc.) as a big, dark, swirling pool around which our life path takes us. The journey is long and sometimes tiring and that pool looks pretty good some times. I find that if I allow myself to take my shoes off and dangle my feet in the waters every once in a while, it can kind of be a little restorative. It also keeps me from jumping in headfirst.
>
> The pool may be a personal comfort now and again, but sitting at its edge gets me nowhere and after a bit, I realize that it doesn't feel all that good to be alone anyway. It helps me come and go to 'the bad place' as I please."[4]

I agree with him. Sometimes I allow myself to spend a whole day being downright angry or sad, which feels good in a naughty way, like scratching a mosquito bite, for the first couple of hours. Then it starts interfering with my life, by making me snappy with my girls, which then takes a long time to undo with apologies and guilt. It also makes it difficult to enjoy things like fine chocolate or seeing a Monarch butterfly in my garden. By the end of the day, feeling this angry or sad is just tiresome and I am done with it.

The "7 Whys" Exercise to Unstick Yourself from Negative Emotions

My father, an engineer, had a great method that he would use to derail some of my more unfeasible requests when I was a young girl. Called the "7 whys," this was a way to show someone, namely me, the irrationality of her or his own emotions or flaws in thinking. Doing a little research reveals that this was an adaptation of a part of a technique called "root cause analysis," developed by Taiichi Ohno, who was the pioneer of the Toyota Production System in the 1950s. He only used 5 whys—I guess my dad just added a couple of "whys" to compensate for the excessive emotions of a young girl, whereas Mr. Ohno was dealing with far more rational and self-controlled Japanese engineers.

Basically, the technique is to ask the question "why?" after a statement. According to Dad's rather bastardized application of the method, if the seventh "why?" yielded anything coherent, then you had something worth discussing. I will spare you some of the humiliating "why?" sequences that originated with my requests for things like horses or a pair of matching Doberman pinschers, but I will tell you that I never got past about four whys before I saw why these things I "needed" did not really fit into our lifestyle.

The same technique can be applied once you get tired of a yucky emotion that is hanging around and getting in your way. It might go something like this:

"I am so angry at everything right now."

Why are you angry? (Why #1)

"Because I have MS."

Why does your MS make you angry? (Why #2)

"Because it makes me feel bad."

Why does feeling bad make you angry? (Why #3)

"Because it is not fair."

Why do you think it is unfair? (Why #4)

"Because I took good care of myself and I got this and it is not my fault. Anyway, other people who don't care anything about taking care of themselves don't have this problem and that pisses me off."

Why are you comparing yourself to other people? (Why #5)

"Because I talked to my friend Amanda today. I am so sick of her talking about how hard things are and being a terrible mother and blaming her son for things that are her fault when she doesn't have any excuse."

Why does that have anything to do with your MS? (Why #6)

"It doesn't. You win."

In sharing this, I am acutely aware that I am not the paragon of maturity or rationality, but our emotions often lead us into places that we would be embarrassed to articulate. The danger is that we often blame it on the MS.

Dabble in Benefit-Finding

Benefit-finding is basically looking for positive results of an adverse thing in one's life: every cloud has a silver lining, always look on the bright side, stuff like that. When it comes to benefit-finding and MS, there seem to be two types of MSers—those who say their MS has been a blessing and those who get violent upon hearing such a statement. Interestingly, research shows that people who are able to see some positive aspects of having MS had improved relationships, more appreciation for life and deepened spirituality.[5] These people also tended to reevaluate priorities, focus more on their families and make positive lifestyle changes.

Like me, you may not be ready to wholeheartedly embrace the idea that MS is a blessing in your life. However, I have reached a place where I can admit that having MS has led me to make some choices that are better for me than the path that I was on. The increasingly aggressive nature of my relapses brought me to the realization that I had to speed up pregnancy so that I could get on a therapy, so I underwent in vitro fertilization, the result of which is my amazing twin girls. I got out of a job in academia that I was ill-suited for and discovered a love of writing. I have been forced to slow down and appreciate the times when I feel, if not good, at least less bad.

The Real World

Be fair to your MS. Don't blame your MS for poor math skills (if you were never good at it), don't blame your MS for marital problems (especially those that would be there anyway). Be fair to your MS and determine what suffering it is causing and what suffering it isn't causing.

I guess the point here is to not blame the MS for all that is not perfect in your life and, in the same vein, give the MS credit where it is due. All that might not outweigh the negative aspects of having MS and all the crappy symptoms that are part of the package, but thinking about it in this way may help release some of the anger if you let it.

The Bottom Line

I will never, ever tell someone that their symptoms are all in their head. I will, however, tell you that I know that even if my symptoms stayed exactly the same, they would feel worse on certain days than on others. What is debilitating on a "sad" day is an annoyance on a happy, busy day. On the days when I get really angry, my fatigue kicks in much earlier and my productive time is much shorter.

This does not mean that we should avoid being sad or angry—as if that is even possible. Sometimes we need to sit down and visit with these emotions. Without looking in the *DSM-IV,* I don't know how angry is "too angry"—is it okay to be mad, but not furious, for instance—or the exact length of time that someone can feel sorry for themselves or anxious before they cross a line. Despite how it might seem at times, I don't think that most of us even get close to being diagnosable as we explore the "dark side." I think it is a necessary part of coping with this disease.

Let's face it—having MS is like living with an abusive roommate who alternates pinching and kicking you with more dramatic things like pushing you down or locking you out of the house in the cold. Except that you can't evict this roommate, can't get the roommate arrested or reprimanded—can't even try to reason with him or her. This can lead to pent-up frustrations and annoyances, which can cycle into destructive feelings that erode self-confidence and hope for the future. Letting off steam and just being angry, sad, lonely, or anxious allows these feelings to find a home rather than buzzing around in your head constantly.

11

Get "In the Mix" for Comfort and Relief

I have a close friend who has been diagnosed with a number of chronic illnesses in the past year—not MS, but similar enough that we can totally relate to each other's trials and tribulations in just getting through the days. Some days the most meaningful, heartfelt exchange that I have comes when I answer the phone and hear a protracted groan in response to my "Hello?" Often, I just whimper or sigh in response, one of us giggles a little and then we hang up. If we both have a little time, we might engage in a good soul-cleansing bitch session about medications, fatigue, headaches, or how our bodies have changed since becoming mothers. We also have plenty of other things in common and we talk about these things, too, but there is something comforting in knowing that I have a "safe place" to tell a real person how I am really feeling.

As people living with multiple sclerosis, many of our struggles are our own and our situations are unique, however, there are many people living with MS out there, experiencing similar fears, challenges, and successes. We watch for new research and treatment developments. We weather disappointments around failed trials or adverse events at the same time. Connecting with others with MS can open up new sources of inspiration and understanding. We can learn from the trials of others, changing our lives for the better.

Are Self-Help Groups for You?

Some people love self-help or support groups, and others really just don't like the whole idea. I get comments from my Internet readers all the time that reflect these differences, along the lines of "I finally went to an MS support group, but I was the only one in a wheelchair and it seemed like everybody already knew each other, so I was uncomfortable and didn't feel welcomed," contrasted with, "I went to a self-help group, but it was a bunch of people in wheelchairs complaining, so I left feeling worse than I did." Of course, I also get the "My MS self-help group has saved my life on more than one occasion and I don't think I could go on without knowing they were there."

Self-help groups have become an integral part of treatment for emotional issues, behavior problems, mental health problems, and for dealing with stressful situations. Many people find that support groups are an invaluable resource for recovery and for empowerment. In the ideal situation, a support group is a group of people who deeply understand each other and can offer practical advice and emotional reinforcement—from the names of good doctors (and those to avoid) to a shoulder to cry on.

Let's start with talking about what self-help groups are. In general, these are groups of people with a similar problem or health condition that come together on a voluntary basis to get support from each other. The idea is that the participants can gain from one another's experiences dealing with the same problems, as well as offer practical advice, strategies, and emotional support. Participants can discuss things that only others with multiple sclerosis could understand and can feel safe when revealing their emotions about this disease. The ultimate desired result of participation in such a group would be renewed self-confidence in dealing with MS, stemming from emotional support and practical directions to take. In the description of support groups on the Web site of the National Multiple Sclerosis Society (NMSS): "Members of self-help groups share a belief that positive personal change happens through individual efforts with the support of others."

In my opinion, one of the reasons that many of us do not find support groups to be right for us is that MS affects such a diverse group of people, and the symptoms and their severity differ drastically between individuals. A twelve-step program is so very effective for some people because, even though all participants are different, they are focused on one goal (abstaining from alcohol, gambling, or drugs, or confronting another problem) using a very specific formula. Thus, all the participants speak a "common language," even though they might be in different stages of recovery.

The Real World

MS is a disease with diversity. There is a variety of symptoms (over 80) and four types of MS, all with different degrees of severity in each individual. Add to that the unique financial and social situations of each person and you end up with quite a few differences between two people with MS.

Although it may work in some cases, a group that is formed around the kernel of multiple sclerosis as the common factor may just be too diverse to work. You could end up with a guy with PPMS in a wheelchair who is seeking legal advice, a young mother with RRMS trying to decide if she should start therapy or continue breastfeeding, a couple of people with mild MS symptoms that want to get the "low-down" on participating in a stem cell clinical trial, and someone who is devastated because he was just reclassified as having SPMS.

Luckily, a lot of people are starting to recognize this and support groups are starting to differentiate across different lines. From the MS Society Web site: "National MS Society self-help groups have different purposes and goals. Groups may focus on support, advocacy, education, or be more social in nature. Some groups also serve specific populations, such as young adults, parents with MS, care partners, or African-Americans."

Make It Better

Don't overlook similarities and what connects you with others amid MS differences.

If you can't find a group that is just right for you, a place where you feel like you are among supportive friends, where you can let your true self shine, there are still plenty of ways to engage with other people with MS. It is important to do this for yourself—whether you connect with them virtually, by telephone, or even by forming your own group, the benefits are worth doing a little digging and extra work. We'll talk about some of the other ways that people with MS maintain contact with each other a little later in the chapter.

Rules of Engagement

Support groups can be great, but this might be a different type of social situation than you are used to. They are basically comprised of strangers (in the beginning) who come together to share pretty personal stuff—things that they may not even tell their families or friends. These strangers may also be seeking emotional support that they are not getting from loved ones. Because many normal steps in a typical "getting to know each other" social process get skipped, it may be wise to strategize the best way to go about things to make sure that you get what you want and need out of these accelerated, "insta-friend" situations.

Consider Social Programs as a Way to Meet People

Maybe you are not ready or interested in a support group, but wouldn't mind meeting other people with MS. Most chapters of the NMSS have some sort of social programs for people living with MS, as well as their friends and families. Some of these have an educational component, but most are just ways to get together and meet people living with similar challenges. There are annual parties, after-hours social meetings at restaurants, and other types of casual mixers. Check with your local chapter.

Think about What You Want from a Support Group

People come to support groups for different reasons. Some come seeking emotional support because they are lonely and feel isolated by living in a world of healthy people who don't "get it." Others are on a mission to find out specific information about how to deal with certain symptoms or medication side effects, or to get a recommendation for a good neurologist. Many are just at a loss and don't know where to go. Then there are some people that just want to be able to be themselves—their tingling, limping, forgetting, fatigued selves—in a crowd that understands, discusses potentially embarrassing problems freely, and even has a couple of much-needed laughs that non-MSers may find macabre or inappropriate.

Get Help

Virtual support includes online chat rooms, discussion groups, forums, and just simple e-mail exchanges that you find value in.

Before you head into a social situation, whether an in-person support group or a virtual meeting place, put some thought into what you want to get out of the group. This will help you find the right forum for you, because you can evaluate different settings and tones of groups easily when you have a personal standard by which you are measuring them. This is not to say that you won't find a group of people that you end up joining and loving, which has nothing to do with your original "wish list." However, you might be able to avoid some disappointment by evaluating things objectively from the outset. For example, if you are seeking support and advice about how to deal with using a wheelchair, a group called "Medical Marijuana for MS Warriors" is probably not an exact fit for your specific need, although you may share some of their ideals and wishes and eventually make this your group of choice.

Think about Who You Want to Be in a Support Group

Take Charge

One of the easiest ways to join a group is to meet a member beforehand for coffee (or even a phone call) and have that person introduce you to the group. That way you get a chance to ask questions before attending to see if the group is a fit, and you already know someone when you arrive. It makes a huge difference.

Yes, we are all people with MS, but in many cases that is not enough of a common thread to ensure that you will automatically click with a particular group right off the bat. Ideally, you will eventually find a group in which you can let it all hang out. Until you are comfortable, however, take some time and watch the dynamics of different groups in order to find your point of entry and the face that you would like to present. For instance, if you are in a support group for newly-diagnosed people who are working through their initial feelings about having MS and struggling with treatment decisions, you may not want to start your introduction by saying things like "anything besides bee venom therapy is for idiots" or "I hate listening to crybabies who are afraid to give themselves injections."

The Real World

Don't feel bad about "shopping" different support groups. You need to find a group that is a good fit for you. If you choose not to be in a group, it is not a judgment on the group, it just means that that group was not right for you at this time in your life.

Think about What Kind of Relationships You Want in a Support Group

To say it is wise to be strategic to get what you need out of a support group may sound calculated and manipulative, but it does not hurt to think about things before you jump in and relationships get established. If you really just want to hear about how others are coping with their anger or sadness, realize that if you announce that you are saving money to go to Costa Rica for stem cell therapy, that topic will become a focus of attention rather than your emotional needs.

Do Your Best

As with anything else, you have to give something to get something. Be prepared to offer emotional and other types of support to fellow group members.

There have been a couple times that I was in a group of people with MS when I really just wanted to enjoy the company of others, but made the mistake of correcting a misconception about MS ("I got the flu last year because MS destroyed my immune system") or throwing out a scientific finding that, although fascinating to me, had no place in the discussion about how hard it is to live with MS on a daily basis. My ill-placed comments distracted from the focus of the conversation, and as a result, my role in the group either became that of someone to answer scientific questions or (more likely) annoying know-it-all to be avoided in the future.

Rules to Get the Most Out of a Group

> *Rule 1. **Be a good listener.*** This might mean biting your tongue if someone says something that you think is wrong or forcing yourself to sit through a really long boring story when you have an excellent anecdote that is much more

appropriate to the situation and could even bring a couple of laughs. You will get your turn to talk.

Rule 2. *Find out the expectations of the group.* If the group members all commit to come on a regular basis and actively participate each time, make sure that you want to do that. Otherwise, you could disrupt the flow and end up not fitting in well.

Rule 3. *Be respectful of others.* This goes beyond general manners of not laughing at someone or not interrupting when it comes to participating in an MS support group. You must remember that we are all on a different journey, and that MS has a different effect on all of us physically, mentally, and emotionally. Never, never compare your situation to others—although someone's tingly feet or occasional tremor may seem trivial in comparison to your reliance on a wheelchair or urinary incontinence, their symptoms are surely a big deal to them. None of us pictured ourselves dealing with any of the crap that MS throws our way, and none of us are "lucky" that we "only" have certain symptoms.

Finding a Support Group

The obvious places to start are the larger MS organizations, such as your local chapter of the National Multiple Sclerosis Society or the Multiple Sclerosis Foundation's self-help directory. Both organizations list the support groups that are affiliated with the organization as well as independent groups that list with the directory. There are a number of groups across the country with delightful names that I would *love* to drop in on, including Pity Us Not Support Group of Central Florida (Leesburg, FL), Wheels & Heels MS Support Group (Pittsburg, KS), MScapaders (Frederick, MD), and The Best Little MS Support Group in Northern New Mexico (Espanola, NM).

Depending on a number of factors, such as the size of your city and the activity level of the MS community there, there may be several groups to choose from. For instance, a huge city like New York City has specific groups for all sorts of different people with MS, including orthodox Jewish women, creative artists, gays and lesbians, people living with MS for 10 years or more, parents, people opting not to take conventional treatment, and children (among others). On the other hand, if you live in a smaller city or town, you may only find one or two groups that are convenient to you. Make sure that you read the description and call the coordinator to find out if this group is right for you. Some groups welcome families and friends, whereas others are just for people with MS. Some provide help with transportation, some meet for lunch, some have speakers come in, some aim to provide an understanding and supportive environment, and many of the descriptions say "come have fun!"

Make It Better

If someone is helpful or you would like to know someone better from you support group, have lunch with them or give them a call. These interactions outside the group setting can be very valuable.

If there is no MS support group in your area or no group that meets your needs, a little bit of digging may reveal groups for people with chronic illnesses or disabilities at your local churches or hospitals. If your search fails to turn up anything of interest to you and you really want to meet other people, consider doing something yourself.

An MS "Salon:" A Fresh Take on Support Groups

So, maybe you've done a little research and can't find a support group in your area. Or maybe you tried it before and got turned off by what you saw as "sitting around complaining in a church basement" and would rather focus on making it a little more uplifting or fun. Maybe you want to focus on MS and only meet with others with MS, or maybe you want to expand your group to include people with other chronic illnesses. Maybe you think it would be great to get together with other men in wheelchairs, other young mothers living with MS, or other people who are considering participating in a clinical trial.

Imagine an MS Salon

Historically, salons were a way for women to increase their education and participation in society, but the definition has been modified to include male hosts. My favorite definition of salon is "a gathering of stimulating people of quality under the guidance of an inspiring host-ess or host, partly to amuse one another and partly to refine their taste and increase their knowledge through conversation."[1]

Make It Better

One of the best examples of a "salon" is the Red Hats Society. These are groups of women over 55 who meet once a month just to have fun. You may have seen them roaming the streets—they all wear red hats and purple outfits. They laugh, are loud, and have a good time. I'm looking forward to joining their ranks someday.

Now, let's take that lovely definition and see how we can apply it to meeting other interesting people who have MS. Salons can be one-time events or recurring events, and can have any imaginable format. The whole point is to find a group comprised of people who you like or would like to get to know better, or people with common interests. It is a way to think outside the support group box and bring together all sorts of people in all sorts of different circumstances to enjoy each others' company.

Some examples of salons might include:

Event salons. These can be gatherings arranged around a one-time event, such as a wine tasting, a special evening at a local restaurant, a tour of area businesses supportive of people with MS, or even just a picnic in a park on a cool day.

Collaborative salons. You can bring together several professionals (for instance, a lawyer, a physician, an accountant) to create a salon to address timely issues for people with MS.

Small salons. A small salon is a great way to get to know people in a small group that gathers on a regular basis. These salons could gather to attend art openings or other cultural events, "tour" restaurants and have dinner together, read and discuss books, or talk about parenting with MS.

Helping salons. These salons can include fundraisers for non-profit organizations or be mentoring salons, where newly-diagnosed people can come to talk to people who have been living with MS for a long time.

Here are some ideas for putting together your own salon:

Choose a topic you love. Find something that you are passionate about and want to share with others. It could be issue-based (advocating for disability rights or access to affordable drugs), cultural (people who love French films, literary clubs), professional (women with MS in the workplace), emotional (divorced people with MS), skill-focused (a creative writing group, people who want to start an MS blog), or other themes (just for fun, dinner clubs). Pick anything that you want to share your passion about.

Brainstorm events. Your salon could simply meet monthly at a cafe near your house or pool money together to buy a box for a baseball game or theater production. Make a list of events and activities that you think would be fun and that others would enjoy. Get your friends together (if you want) and brainstorm ideas that get you all really excited.

Do Your Best

Start your group with three friends. You can share the planning and advertising work. In the worst case, you'll have a group of four people who like to get together.

Let other people know about it. Choose an event to do, work out the logistics, write up some good descriptions, and figure out where to advertise. You can talk to people in existing support groups, see about putting a notice in a local paper, or talk to your local MS Society chapter about advertising to their members. Maybe you could hand out flyers at a local MS walk. If you choose to make it a recurring event, the Multiple Sclerosis Foundation may include you in their support group directory, as well.

Meet the MS Community From the Comfort of Your Own Home

There are lots of reasons that many of us like to interact with other MSers from home. Maybe there is no support group within a convenient distance from your home, or maybe it is difficult for you to get out because of symptoms, disabilities, or difficulties driving. Perhaps you are not ready to sit in a room with other people with MS in an unstructured support atmosphere, and you prefer discussing very specific topics with anonymous people. Regardless of your reasons, topics of interest, and style of communication, there is a whole world of virtual "friends" waiting to meet you and offer, as well as receive, much-needed support, advice, and new ideas.

Take Charge

The Internet can be great, but you do need to balance your "screen time" with other activities. Be a bit goal-oriented, set time limits, and don't stay on the computer so long that you feel weird rejoining real life.

Health researchers have looked into why people use online support sites and found that the people that were the most active on these sites loved things like convenience and access to information, but they also liked the ability to ask advice and the lack of embarrassment when dealing with personal issues. Studies found that many people perceived improvements in their quality of life and reported that their health complaints or symptoms were less severe after they joined the site. On the other hand, there are some health professionals that point to evidence that too much time in the virtual world can lead to isolation and depression, especially if it is at the expense of socializing with friends.

Special Rules for Participating in an Online Group to Get the Most Out of It

Rule 1. Open up. You are anonymous when online, so you can be more open and free with your opinions and feelings. Use this situation wisely—express feelings that you have been keeping bottled up, share embarrassing experiences, let out your frustrations.

Rule 2. Pause a moment. Think before you type and reread posts before you send them to ensure that you are not inadvertently offending someone and that you are communicating what you intend to.

Rule 3. Guard your identity. Be cautious, even paranoid, about sharing personal information—don't post telephone numbers and don't use e-mail addresses comprised of your full name.

The Real World

When a jerk is harassing you in a forum (and there will be at least one), my favorite strategy is to thank them. Not only is it classy, but it takes all the fun out of tormenting you, which usually results in the person leaving you alone. Just something slightly tongue-in-cheek, like "Thank you so much for your thoughtful insights," can take the air out of anyone's mean sails.

Rule 4. Cool down. Don't respond immediately to a post or message that has offended or angered you. Reread it a couple of times and realize that people often have a difficult time communicating accurately in writing, or may not understand "netiquette," such as ALL CAPS MEANS THAT YOU ARE SHOUTING. Even if you do decide that the poster has truly intended to tell you that you are stupid, for example if they type, "I cannot believe how very stupid you are," think before you answer. I have found that drowning a mean person in virtual honey often serves me better than going on the attack, because others feel free to participate in the discussion and often my supporters come to my defense.

Take Charge

If you find you are wasting precious energy worried about how people responded to your message or trying to think up ways to change someone's mind in a debate, it may be time to leave that forum. Life is too short to bring negative energy from the Internet into it.

Forums and Message Boards

A forum is an interesting way to "talk" to other MSers and find answers to specific questions. There are lots of forums out there for people with MS, but I am going to mention a couple to get you started, depending on what type of information or virtual environment you are looking for:

MSWorld (www.msworld.org/forum) As of this writing, MSWorld has over 30,000 members and over 80,000 threads (topics) under which messages are posted. It is well-organized and pretty easy to navigate if you are new to the forum scene. It covers many different aspects of living with MS and has boards specifically geared toward young people, women only, men only, seniors, and people with progressive forms of MS. MSWorld has some other cool things going on, like teleconferences that you can submit questions to before the event, which then get turned into podcasts. Go to www.mscast.net for the schedule or to hear the podcasts.

BrainTalk (brain.hastypastry.net) and NeuroTalk (neurotalk.psychcentral.com) both offer MS information and support in a similar format, but are smaller communities. As such, it seems like the people know each other better, which can be great if you want to take the effort to get to know other people and join a true community, but intimidating for people new to forum participation.

The Real World

Many of the major MS pharmaceutical companies also sponsor community areas for people with MS, as well as virtual and in-person "educational" sessions. These can be great, just be aware that the purpose of the company is to promote its therapy.

This is MS (www.thisisms.com/forums.html) This is MS describes itself as "an unbiased, unaffiliated site dedicated to eradicating Multiple Sclerosis." As such it encourages members to post information on all MS treatments, both approved and in trial, as well as alternative approaches like low-dose naltrexone, Aimspro, and diet regimens. The forum is well-organized, with individual boards for many of the current treatments and some of those in the pipeline. These boards are further broken down into many subtopics under each one. There are also forums about living with MS, but really this is the place to come to find out "what the deal is" with treatments and see how many of these scientific findings are likely to affect our daily lives eventually.

Disaboom While not specifically for people with MS, Disaboom (www.disaboom.com) is an amazing place for anybody with a chronic illness or disability to connect with others. There is a very active forum, members can create their own blogs on the site, and there are chat rooms. One of the most intriguing features of the site is the virtual "groups" of people with different interests—disabled surfers, people needing chronic pain control, crafters with disabilities, adaptive skiers, and people with service dogs can all find virtual friends with similar interests here.

Webpals

These are the modern-day version of pen pals, using the Internet and e-mail. It works by people posting a little information about themselves and the types of things they would like to talk about, as well as what kind of person they would like to discuss these things with. There is minimal moderation, in that you initially answer your webpal through the "host" of the service, who forwards your message to the person. If they are interested, they will write back to you directly, and you are on your own to exchange messages as often as you like. The best site for this is "Webpals" at Jooly's Joint (www.webpals.org), which operates this service free of charge. Jooly's Joint MS Pride is a special place for gay men and lesbians who are living with MS to find one another.

Make It Better

Make a pledge to try to reach out to others in at least three different ways. Find others with MS. Make a connection.

Blog It

It has been shown that writing about traumatic experiences actually has healing properties. I don't know if the theory applies to the extent that a heartfelt outpouring of emotions about symptoms or injections onto your computer screen would make any difference that could be seen on an MRI image, but it might be just the catharsis you need to get through a rough patch. "Blog" is short for "weblog" and is a loose term for a site that is maintained with regular entries of personal essays, news, or other kinds of commentary. There are many, many MSers out there who maintain blogs. Check out the Carnival of MS Bloggers (carnivalofms-bloggers.blogspot.com), which is a compilation of over 100 blogs, to give you inspiration. You can also consider creating and maintaining a page on Facebook (www.facebook.com), which gives you a little more control over what parts of your site people have access to.

Calls

Sometimes it is easier to talk about difficult issues with someone who you don't know and can't see. I may have been taken off the list from telemarketers and fundraisers because there have been times that I have picked up the phone and actually answered their opening question of "How are you doing this afternoon, ma'am?" with the actual truth—my head hurt, I couldn't feel my feet, and I was dreading my injection. A much healthier and more fruitful alternative would have been to hook up with one of these amazing programs in which a volunteer with MS calls to chat, check in on you, or give you updates as to what is happening in the world of MS research. The Multiple Sclerosis Association of America (MSAA) has "Reassurance Calls," and the Multiple Sclerosis Foundation's (MSF) program is called "We Care, We Call." You can sign up for MSF's program by calling 1-888-673-6287 or contact them by e-mail at support@msfocus.org. You may schedule a call to happen monthly, weekly, or every couple of days.

MSFriends (msfriends.org) offers the first telephone helpline staffed with people who have MS. The helpline at 1-866-MSFRIENDS (1-866-673-7436) is staffed 24 hours a day, 7 days a week. The trained volunteers operate under the principle of "friends helping friends" to provide specific information about MS as well as emotional support.

Teleconference Self-help/Support Groups.

Some self-help groups also offer teleconference self-help groups. These include Cafe con Leche: Conversation and Support for People Living with MS (in Spanish), MS and Cancer Telephone Self-Help Group, and Home Is Your Range Self-Help Group. Check with your chapter of the National Multiple Sclerosis Society or call the main office at 1-800-344-4867, to find out more.

Find and Use Resources

Over the years, I have been involved with a number of organizations that had the mission to help others—the staff of these organizations spent endless hours writing grants, designing programs, printing educational materials, doing research among their constituents—all with the mission to make people's lives a little better, whether these were people living with HIV/AIDS, young women involved in the sex trade in Moscow, or the parents of disabled children.

What do you think the biggest challenge was for these organizations? Of course, there was never enough money to do every program and it was hard to find staff that was both qualified and willing to work for not-for-profit level salaries. Yet the very biggest problem of these organizations was reaching their constituents—in other words, actually finding and connecting with the very people that they were in the business of helping. It is the same way for services for people with multiple sclerosis. There are vast resources, both human and financial, devoted to making life easier or better for us somehow. It is our job to find these people and programs and help them help us.

Make It Better

Nothing is more disheartening to MS support organizations than having a lot of resources and no people showing up to use them. Go to the talks, accept the services, and create a demand.

Below is an overview of some of the many, many types of resources available to people living with multiple sclerosis. Please check the Internet for updated contact information and additional programs.

Helplines

Helplines are run by various organizations and dedicated to helping people with MS access the resources they provide or hooking people up with local services. For instance, the helpline of the National Multiple Sclerosis Society (NMSS) at 1-800-344-4867 can provide help locating clinics, neurologists, clinical trials, and updates on research progress. The MSF helpline (1-888-673-6287) is answered by caseworkers and peer counselors who tailor support to each person's needs.

Information

Clearly, there is a huge amount of information available to people with MS. For people who like to read books, both The Multiple Sclerosis Association of America (MSAA) and the local chapters of the National Multiple Sclerosis Society (NMSS) have lending libraries. Both organizations have extensive online compilations of articles that you can read on screen or print out.

Web Sites

There are many, many Web sites geared towards sharing information about MS. I wanted to highlight a couple of interesting ones to illustrate the diversity of what is out there.

ChronicBabe. Geared towards young women with chronic illnesses, this site (www.chronicbabe.com) is pretty fun, as well as being informative. As explained by the founder and editrix, "this site caters to the younger Babes because there just isn't a lot of good information available on how to be young, wild, creative, sexy and daring while managing a complicated health regimen. The challenges for younger women are unique, and we deserve a resource all our own." In addition to the well-written articles on the site (click on the little speech bubble in the upper right hand corner that says "psssst!" for some great articles about sex), my favorite section is called "Beautiful Things," which has online shopping for things like jeweled syringe cases, pretty beaded medical alert bracelets, and crutches that actually resemble fashion accessories. ChronicBabe has also launched a podcast series of educational discussions and interviews with experts. All you women out there, give it a try—I listened to the one called *ChronicBabe 101: The "First Four Steps."* No kidding, I felt like I was hanging out chatting with a cool friend (and we could all use more of those).

Myelin Repair Foundation. This is a fascinating organization. As you will learn from their site (www.myelinrepair.org), The Myelin Repair Foundation is actually "the only non-profit medical research foundation solely focused on identifying myelin repair drug targets that will lead to treatments for multiple sclerosis." As such, it provides fascinating information about this area of MS research, including very technical scientific research reports and white papers.

Accelerated Cure Project. The Accelerated Cure Project for Multiple Sclerosis is also a scientifically-geared organization, which is "dedicated to curing multiple sclerosis" by determining the cause of MS. It has developed a framework for accomplishing this noble task, called "The Cure Map," which details procedures and progress in uncovering some of the mysteries surrounding MS. My favorite thing about this organization is "The Accelerated Cure Project MS Repository," which is a collection of biological samples and data from people with MS (you can be one of them) and their relatives. Without going into too much detail (you can find this info on the site), these samples and data are made accessible to scientists, as long as they share their findings with each other—this is a fabulous example of the kind of collaboration that needs to take place around research. The site (www.acceleratedcure.org) is full of detailed articles about different aspects of MS, ranging from discussions of neuroanatomy to reviews of popular MS books to an overview of the American health-care market as it affects people with MS. All of the issues of the newsletter are archived. The site also hosts MSNews (msnews.acceleratedcure.org), which is described as "a daily newspaper of 'what's up in Multiple Sclerosis' with an interactive letters to the editor attached to each story" and contains current information about advances in research.

Magazines

Check out *Momentum*, the monthly publication of the NMSS; *Multiple Sclerosis Quarterly Report (MSQR)*; *The Motivator*, MSAA's quarterly magazine; Rocky Mountain MS center newsletter; *MSFocus*, published quarterly by MSF; *Mobility Plus*; *Keep S'myelin*; and the print newsletter from Accelerated Cure Project.

Online Educational Videos

MSAA offers a fairly large collection of online videos (www.msassociation .org/programs/videos) covering medical, lifestyle, and legal aspects of MS.

Wellness and Exercise Programs

Different chapters of the NMSS provide wellness programs designed with the needs of MSers in mind. Programs differ by chapter, but include aquatics, art therapy, dance, Make Your Mark Day, physical training, Pilates, Pi-Yo, Tai Chi, therapeutic horseback riding, yoga, and Yo Tai. Programs are free unless otherwise noted.

Career Planning and Employment Resources

MS Workplace (msworkplace.com), a joint venture of Monster and NMSS, is a Web site that is "the first-of-its-kind online initiative that provides MS-specific career advice, workplace tips, and job postings for the MS community." It also has information for employers of people with MS.

Life Coaching

MSAA offers group "life coaching" sessions to people with MS via telephone and online. Some areas of focus will include the following: adjustment to living with MS, health and wellness issues, stress management, work/life balance, family relationships, medication adherence issues, self advocacy, help finding resources, behavioral approaches to pain management, and planning for the future.

Know Your Stuff

SSDI and SSI are mechanisms through which the Social Security Administration can assist people living with disability; resources include monthly payments to help with living costs.

Legal Advice

Different forms of legal assistance are available in different regions, and many can be found or accessed through the NMSS. Many of these services focus on helping people with SSDI and SSI claims, including people who want to apply, those who have applied, and those who have been denied and wish to appeal. Other services may include assistance with long term care planning, including wills, medical directives, or power of attorney, as well as domestic issues, such as divorce or custody disputes. There are also legal services to address employment issues, including matters covered by the Americans with Disabilities Act, such as job discrimination or job accommodation. Chapter staff may direct you to the right community resources or make a referral to an attorney who is has experience with MS and disability issues who may be able to provide a pro-bono consult.

Financial Planning and Assistance

The NMSS has started a program called "Money Matters" to provide expertise to individuals with MS, both for people needing immediate financial advice as well as those who are planning for the future. Professional financial advisors offer money management and related financial education including simple budgeting skills, managing cash flow, and debt repayments, as well as general financial planning services. They can also assist with more specific issues such as insurance analysis, claims assistance, and employee benefit analysis, as well as long-term planning, such as retirement planning and estate planning. For more information call 1-800-344-4867.

The NMSS also provides emergency financial assistance for individuals facing an immediate financial crisis or who are not able to obtain the basic needs of food, utilities, or shelter. They also offer summer emergency assistance for MSers with heat intolerance who need help in the months from June to September. For more information call 1-800-344-4867.

MRIs Paid For

The MRI Diagnostic Fund of the MSAA helps individuals obtain an initial diagnostic MRI of the brain, and the MRI Institute will help with other MRIs by working with MS centers, imaging centers, and doctors' offices. In cases of insurance denials or non-insured individuals, MSAA can also assist with payment for a diagnostic MRI. Call 1-800-532-7667 for more information.

Help Getting Your Home Modified and Staying Mobile

Some NMSS chapters have programs to provide services and goods to people who have needs not met by other community resources. According to the description of one chapter's program, "Provision of services must either maintain or enhance: 1. Dignity in managing the symptoms of MS; 2. Independence and safety in the performance of daily tasks; and 3. Mobility within the community." Please note that the requirements and services or assistance provided by each chapter vary, so it is best to call your local chapter for specifics. There is also information about accessible transportation on chapter Web sites.

MSF also has an Assistive Technology (AT) Program, which "strives to educate and assist individuals with MS across the country about the myriad of AT options available and how to access these options." This program may help you locate a specific product, or even provide or give funding to help you purchase devices such as communication aids, computers, orthotics, home and vehicle modifications, or mobility aids.

The MSAA Equipment Distribution Program "offers clients an extensive inventory of products designed to improve their safety, dignity, mobility, and independence. MSAA provides these products at no charge and ships directly to the client."

Help Getting Cooling Products

The MSF Cooling Program offers a variety of items free of charge, including cooling vests, neckties, wristbands, bandanas, work collars, skull-pads, and baseball hats. The Multiple Sclerosis Association of America (MSAA) also has a cooling equipment distribution program that provides special cooling apparel at no charge to people with MS.

Homecare Assistance

The MSF Home Care Assistance Grant Program helps link up people with MS to appropriate local services. If these types of resources are not available in a region, direct support will be provided on a temporary basis through the MSF Home Care Assistance Grant Program. Available services include home care (such as personal hygiene services, light housekeeping, grocery shopping, meal preparation, and transportation to and from appointments); therapy visits with an occupational, physical, or speech therapist; short-term respite care by a properly trained individual; and assistance transitioning home from the hospital.

Retreats and Camps

The Heuga Center (www.heuga.org) runs the CAN DO Program, which is a retreat comprised of individualized consultations, lectures, and workshops that emphasize general health, physical fitness, and psychological well-being. The programs address lifestyle strategies that include exercise, nutrition, self-management, social interaction, and support for the person with MS and their support partners.

The various NMSS chapters also run a variety of camps for people with MS and their relatives, including Camp Can Do (different from that run by the Heuga Center) for people living with MS who require assistance with everyday tasks (Texas), Camp Hope (Arizona) for children ages 8 to 15 living with a family member with MS, and MS Mountain Getaway (Southern California) for people with MS and their spouses.

Cruise for a Cause

MSF runs a yearly one-week cruise for people with MS and their caregivers. The cruise features support group meetings, talks by neurologists and researchers, and accessible shore excursions. The itineraries vary and include routes through the Caribbean and Alaska.

For Caregivers

Some chapters of the MS Society provide respite care or vouchers for respite care so that caregivers can get a break.

Accessible Housing

MSAA owns and operates five barrier-free apartment complexes in New Jersey and North Carolina that provide accessible, affordable housing for physically disabled adults in an independent living environment. Rent is subsidized through the government, so that rental payments are 30% of a tenant's adjusted gross income.

The Bottom Line

There is no question about it. Multiple sclerosis is a very lonely disease, even if we are surrounded by helpful and understanding people who love us. There are no words to describe many of the symptoms that we have, but most of us are usually plagued by one symptom or another at any given time and end up self-editing everything that we say or do in order not to appear whiny or needy or anything but perfectly fine to those around us.

Get Help

There are lots of reasons to connect with other people with MS, but one of the best reasons is to gain a little bit of perspective. We are not alone, others have gone before us, and we will get through it (somehow).

It seems that for many of us, meeting other people with multiple sclerosis, whether in person or virtually, would be like having a cozy little clubhouse where we were exclusive members. I frequently get e-mail messages from other people with multiple sclerosis, usually asking questions about an article that I have written or asking me to defend something that I have said about one of the MS drugs. My favorite messages are the ones that say, "Thank you for letting me know I am not alone in my anger about MS," or "I never knew that other people had the MS hug as bad as I do," or "You summed it up when you said if non-MSers felt like we did on one of our 'good days,' they would call in sick to work."

It is comments like these that remind me that there are others suffering alone out there, when what we really need to do is get together and be able to laugh about things that might otherwise make us cry, and cry about things that no one else would understand.

12

Make Things Better

As a person living with MS, I find that almost every day has a particular struggle to work through or an obstacle to overcome that probably wouldn't come up for a healthy person. Some of these things I deal with by reclassifying them as annoyances rather than problems, and I just muster through the best that I can. I reassure myself that it really is okay if the neighborhood meeting is held outside at noon in 90-degree weather—I didn't want to participate, anyway. Or I might expend a good deal of mental energy wondering if I will actually feel good enough to make it through a conference that I should attend, given that there don't seem to be many chances or places to rest and that I will be expected to participate in scientific discussions throughout the day, despite fatigue and cognitive dysfunction issues. I decide that I won't really be able to perform up to snuff, so I recommend that someone else goes, even though I was pretty excited about some of the topics.

So it goes, day after day, for many of us. We make up excuses, we feign disinterest, we withdraw a little. At some point, however, there just has to be a "no," maybe even a "NO!" It may be a seemingly-insignificant moment that changes your views on life and what is right for you. One such moment came for me back when I had just finished college and I was learning how to function in the real world. I had seen a doctor for what I am now pretty sure was MS-related depression, and he promptly prescribed a medication that was all over the media: Prozac. I went to get my prescription filled at a local pharmacy, literally trembling with all the embarrassment and nervousness that could be embodied in a young woman who is just starting to find out that many things in life, but especially herself, are not perfect. The guy behind the pharmacy counter barely looked at me when I approached to pick up my prescription, instead yelling from 15 feet away, "Yeah, what was that for again?" I stood there silent and mortified, unable and unwilling to respond. He said, "You gonna tell me what you need, or what?" A switch flipped in me from humiliation to fury. I got angry—angry for myself and my embarrassment, but also angry for all the people that might also feel too stigmatized to answer this punky idiot. So I answered, loudly saying, "Yeah, dude, I'll tell you what I need. Let's start with some lithium and some AZT, throw in the morning-after pills and some antibiotics for my raging gonorrhea. Oh yeah, I also need some Valium with that. Got any methadone back there? Most of all, don't forget my *Prozac*!" I would never want to see a video of myself at that moment, but when I relive it, I mostly remember how good it felt to say, "Enough is enough."

Make It Better

If we all agree to make things better whenever we can, our worlds—both individually and as a member of the community of people with MS—will slowly, but steadily, improve.

Being your own advocate means standing up for yourself by understanding your rights and fighting for them. It means figuring out what is right for you or what you need, then making sure that you get it. In order to be your own best advocate, you may have to turn your preconceived ideas of authority upside down. You have to remember that you are the expert in terms of what you need, and you need to eliminate notions that others know better or that the system is impossible to navigate or that things are too hard to change.

You can change from a passive patient to an active advocate for your own health care and your rights as a person living with MS. The things that will make you an active advocate are simple, but not easy for everyone to do. You will have to examine personal assumptions about authority figures and health care that are still deeply ingrained in the culture. You will learn that you can, indeed, be your own advocate.

Universal Approaches to Advocacy, or How to Get What You Want

Many people associate advocacy with hand-lettered signs and lots of screaming about volatile issues, which get covered on the evening news—biased toward one extreme position or another. Advocacy, though, is simply the act of speaking up in an attempt to change things for the better, whether it is just for yourself in a particular situation, or for a larger group.

Regardless of whether you are trying to get something done that you need or trying to tackle a problem for the greater good, there are some keys to increasing your chances of success.

Rule 1. Define your problem precisely and be very specific about what you want to change.

I can remember a time a couple of years ago when my neuro came into the exam room with his usual concerned smile. The ratio of smile to concern reversed when I tearfully said, "I feel like crap, utter crap. Please fix it," and proceeded to plant my face onto the edge of his desk because I felt too tired to hold my head up, and maybe a little for dramatic effect. That appointment devolved into a kind of organic counseling session about the unpredictability of MS, during which I caught him looking at me in a way that told me he was trying to determine whether I was depressed or just distraught. Of course, he reviewed my recent MRI, asked me all the usual questions, and conducted a neurological exam, which pretty much showed that I had not really progressed on the disability scale, and that my MS was pretty stable from the year before. I left with no solutions, just the reassurance that I wasn't having a relapse.

Take Charge

No one can help you make a difference unless you know what you want. Avoid wasting your (and others') time by just venting or expressing the injustice of things. Have a clearly defined goal when you seek change.

Contrast that with the time that I went in with a precise description of my fatigue and how it was affecting my life. I spent some time thinking about the appointment before going in and answered the questions outlined in "How to talk to your doctor about your symptoms" in Chapter 3. I told him that my fatigue was making it very difficult to take care of my toddlers, and that I woke up feeling terrible, with a fatigue that not only affected my thinking, but that was accompanied by nausea and headaches. I let him know that I was not expecting miracles and that I would be happy with just "better"—my lifestyle at that moment would allow me to take a short nap at noon when I put the girls down. I also told him that I would rather be a little more conservative in my approach with medications and would trade getting less energy from my meds to avoid the potential side effects of anxiety or a jittery feeling. I left with a prescription for a disabled placard and a lowish-dose prescription for Provigil, with the plan to check back in three months to see if I wanted to continue on this med or try something else. I was also told to call sooner if I was still experiencing the same level of fatigue in a month. I left feeling proud and in control, despite my fatigue.

Rule 2. Have a well-researched solution to offer.

In your desire to make something in your life better, you may get emotional and make assumptions that people know what to do to help you. For instance, you may decide that your job is too physically demanding, even though you love it. Going to your boss and crying, "it's just too hard, I can't keep up, but please don't fire me," does not give him much to work with and puts him in an awkward situation. On the other hand, outlining different ideas for adjusting your schedule (such as allowing you to work from home on specific projects) or making modifications to your work space or the way that you do things shows that the job means something to you and that you want to work something out.

Know Your Stuff

Knowing the options will often prevent you from making mistakes or pursuing the wrong path. A bit of research before seeking a solution can save time, effort, and money.

Likewise, telling your doctor that you *cannot stand* the spasticity in your leg anymore and giving the simple directive to make it feel better right away sends the message that this is your priority above all else. He may skip over some of the more conservative approaches like physical therapy or oral medications and go straight for something like intrathecal baclofen in an attempt to relieve your distress. You may be unprepared, however, for the idea of surgery to implant the pump, or the fact that the pump will be visible under your skin, or the potential side effects of fatigue from this drug. Some consequences of not communicating precisely might include wasting time that could have been used to solve your problem with more conservative measures or, more dramatically, you may end up taking actions that you end up regretting.

Rule 3. Figure out who can solve your problem, then focus on that specific decision maker.

In some cases it probably *seems* very clear whom you are trying to influence and who has access to what you need to make things better for yourself. When you are trying to deal with a symptom medically, a logical target seems to be your doctor. When you have decided that adjusting your work schedule to allow for "flex time" would help you cope with your fatigue, you would no doubt start by talking to your immediate supervisor. When you want to get permission to install some safety features in your rental apartment, it would seem like the building superintendent would be the person to take care of that sort of thing.

However, when you are going after what you want, make sure you take the time and think things through all the way. Remember, most people operate within a hierarchical structure and it might take a couple of tries and some patience to find out who holds the keys to resolving your problem. For instance, your doctor might need to get a procedure pre-approved from your insurance company before proceeding, your immediate supervisor will probably need to get approval from someone higher up in the company before granting your request, and your building's superintendent will most likely need to get proposed changes to the property approved by a landlord.

Do Your Best

Sure, we are angry, but when advocating for change we need to make allies, not enemies. Evoke sympathy and help people help us.

Be patient as you climb up the ladder in an attempt to fix your issue. It helps to put yourself in the place of the person you are dealing with at each step and realize that most people really just don't want to get in trouble and want to do things with the least amount of stress to themselves as possible. Think back to times that you may have gotten upset about things and attacked the first person that had to tell you bad news—you may end up screaming at the customer service representative at your phone company for an overcharge, it may have been that the line at airport security was too long and you missed your plane so you let loose on the guy checking identification and boarding passes, it may be that your insurance company denied payment for a medication and you give the pharmacist an earful about it. Not only were these people most likely not able to help solve your problem, you probably alienated someone who might have been helpful in getting you in front of the right person or finding an alternative solution. I know I have learned this lesson the hard way, and probably not for the last time—although I now try my best to fight the urge to take out my frustration on the first person standing in my way.

Rule 4. Be assertive and confident, not aggressive and combatant, in your communications.

While advocacy is fighting to get what you want, the method behind the "fight" might not look like any fight you've ever seen (or fought). Standing up for yourself is an act of preserving and pursuing dignity— as such, it should be done in a dignified manner.

People who are assertive and confident seem to be in control— they are folks who are going to get what they want because it is right, because it is how the world should work. People listen to those individuals who can present their views in a way that makes everything they say come across as objective fact, thus it is more likely that people will work to help them.

In order to come across as authoritative, but likeable, a couple of things need to be kept in mind. Most importantly, stay calm and cool. Never insult or threaten the other person, that makes people focus on themselves (and their feelings of anger at you), while taking their attention away from your problem. It is important to stick to the topic that you are discussing and not let emotions take you into other territory of other, unrelated issues. You can ask the other person if you are communicating clearly (this is kind of a trick to reset them and make sure that they are getting the message)—I often say something such as, "You know, I appreciate your time. This is so important to me that I just want to make sure that my emotions are not interfering with what I want to say. Have you understood what I said so far, or have I left out something?" Listen carefully when the other person talks. Ask the other person to clarify their point or repeat important information.

Rule 5. Keep notes and track your progress.

My dad has a spiral-bound notebook in which he records every detail of his life. It is organized chronologically, so that the entries appear almost schizophrenic in their lack of relation to each other besides occurring in sequence. A page may have a series of entries: "11:47 am conversation with Dr. Godfrey, LDL cholesterol 120, HDL 57 doc says fine yes stay on Lipitor; 12:48 pm Jack Murray (contractor's new asst) came to look at drainage ditch says at least a week (not per our agreement) to finish water still standing not happy will call Jack and complain maybe compromise possible will not ask him to fix gutter need new guy; 1:32 pm recipe for spinach with sesame seeds on food network boil spinach 3 minutes and mix with 2 tsp sesame seeds and 1 tsp sesame oil probably use baby spinach."

Do Your Best

If you don't write it down and can't remember important details, it is like it never happened.

Whether you are talking to your neurologist, your insurance company, or a lawyer, it is important to be able to present your facts. Consider these two exchanges:

"Hi, I hope you can help me out. On November 2nd of this year, I spoke with Anne Butler in customer service about the refusal of payment for my MRI of the brain and cervical spine that I received on September 30th. She told me that it was a matter of the wrong diagnostic code entered in the form submitted by my neurologist office and that it did not reflect that this MRI was conducted because my neurologist thought that I was having a relapse, rather than a routine MRI. That is the reason that the September 30th MRI occurred less than two months after my annual MRI, which I got on August 7th. I called my neurologist's office the same day that I spoke with Ms. Butler and explained the situation. They pulled up the record and saw their error, which they promised to rectify that same day and resubmit the form by fax. Has that been resolved and when can I expect to receive notice that my account is now clear?"

Compare this to:

"Yeah, I just got another big bill from you guys. I called there about a month or two ago and talked to a lady that said my doctor's office screwed up and that you guys weren't going to pay unless they fixed it. I called my doctor's office and they said it's your fault, and I am not going to pay $1,700 for a stupid MRI that I didn't even want. So are you going to take care of this or should I sue you?"

Take Charge

Use people's names. Thank them, by name, and take the time to remember their names. It makes a huge difference in getting someone to go the extra mile to solve your problem. It also informs them that you are paying attention and know whom to blame if something goes wrong or if they give you incorrect information.

The types of details that you will want to write down include the time and date of the conversation, the name and title of the person you spoke with, and what they said (what they told you to do, what the problem was, what they promised to do). In addition, you should write down what you said to them, especially what you said you would do. You should also make sure to take notes of specific follow-up items— whom should you contact, as well as when and how (letter, fax, e-mail, by phone) you should contact this person, or if someone will be contacting you, who that person is, when, and how).

Rule 6. Put it all together and go after what you want.

In most cases, you can get what you want if you go about it the right way. In other cases, you can at least make things better, even if the outcome is not exactly what you envisioned. Applying these ideals and techniques to any interaction of consequence will ensure that you have laid the groundwork for the best possible solution. You will not have to clean up any messes in order to keep moving forward. Everything will be clean and logical, calm, and dignified. You will allow people to help you and let them feel good about doing it.

A Brief Intro to the History of the Disability Movement

Since my MS diagnosis, whenever I leave my familiar surroundings, there is a part of me that is constantly maintaining an inner monologue about what sights I could see or activities I could or could not easily do if my mobility becomes severely compromised. Sure, I could see that show if I was in a wheelchair—if I didn't mind sitting in the "nosebleed" section, arriving first and leaving last. I *guess* I could navigate that subway in a scooter, if I knew exactly which exits had elevator access and where the cars came close enough to the platform to eliminate the gap where wheels could get stuck. The reality is that, for many people, accessibility is fairly difficult and requires much advance planning—and usually some last-minute detours. In many foreign countries, it is simply out of the question. There remains much to be done.

Despite the current challenges and "wish list" items still outstanding, we have come a long, long way in the effort to integrate people with disabilities into society.

Take a moment and try to imagine the following scene: The setting is 1977 in a federal office building in San Francisco. The country had witnessed a couple of decades of the civil rights movement, so people were pretty used to seeing protests and acts of civil disobedience, especially in the liberal, outspoken Bay Area. But hold on here—zoom in a moment and take a closer look at this group of over 100 people demanding their rights. There are people in wheelchairs, deaf folks, blind people, people who are developmentally disabled, and people hooked up to portable respirators—and they are *pissed off.*

What this group wanted was that any entity that received federal monies make buildings, transportation, and services accessible to people with disabilities in compliance with Section 504 of the 1973 Rehabilitation Act, four years after it was signed. Although there were similar demonstrations taking place across the country, most fizzled after a few days. In contrast, the San Francisco demonstrators hunkered down and stayed in place for almost four weeks, making it the longest occupation of federal property on record to date. The protesters won their battle on April 28, 1977, when HEW Secretary Joseph Califano endorsed the regulations and signed it into law.

On July 26, 1990, President George H. W. Bush signed into law the Americans with Disabilities Act (ADA) saying these words, "Let the shameful wall of exclusion finally come tumbling down." Though not perfect, the law is impressive. For an eloquent description of the rather dismal state of affairs involving rights for people with disabilities less than two decades ago, read the "Findings" section of the ADA below:

The Congress finds that

(1) some 43,000,000 Americans have one or more physical or mental disabilities, and this number is increasing as the population as a whole is growing older;

(2) historically, society has tended to isolate and segregate individuals with disabilities, and, despite some improvements, such forms of discrimination against individuals with disabilities continue to be a serious and pervasive social problem;

(3) discrimination against individuals with disabilities persists in such critical areas as employment, housing, public accommodations, education, transportation, communication, recreation, institutionalization, health services, voting, and access to public services;

(4) unlike individuals who have experienced discrimination on the basis of race, color, sex, national origin, religion, or age, individuals who have experienced discrimination on the basis of disability have often had no legal recourse to redress such discrimination;

(5) individuals with disabilities continually encounter various forms of discrimination, including outright intentional exclusion, the discriminatory effects of architectural, transportation, and communication barriers, overprotective rules and policies, failure to make modifications to existing facilities and practices, exclusionary qualification standards and criteria, segregation, and relegation to lesser services, programs, activities, benefits, jobs, or other opportunities;

(6) census data, national polls, and other studies have documented that people with disabilities, as a group, occupy an

inferior status in our society, and are severely disadvantaged socially, vocationally, economically, and educationally;

(7) individuals with disabilities are a discrete and insular minority who have been faced with restrictions and limitations, subjected to a history of purposeful unequal treatment, and relegated to a position of political powerlessness in our society, based on characteristics that are beyond the control of such individuals and resulting from stereotypic assumptions not truly indicative of the individual ability of such individuals to participate in, and contribute to, society;

(8) the Nation's proper goals regarding individuals with disabilities are to assure equality of opportunity, full participation, independent living, and economic self-sufficiency for such individuals; and

(9) the continuing existence of unfair and unnecessary discrimination and prejudice denies people with disabilities the opportunity to compete on an equal basis and to pursue those opportunities for which our free society is justifiably famous, and costs the United States billions of dollars in unnecessary expenses resulting from dependency and nonproductivity.

Now, read what Congress wants to do about it:

It is the purpose of this chapter

(1) to provide a clear and comprehensive national mandate for the elimination of discrimination against individuals with disabilities;

(2) to provide clear, strong, consistent, enforceable standards addressing discrimination against individuals with disabilities;

(3) to ensure that the Federal Government plays a central role in enforcing the standards established in this chapter on behalf of individuals with disabilities; and

(4) to invoke the sweep of congressional authority, including the power to enforce the fourteenth amendment and to regulate commerce, in order to address the major areas of discrimination faced day-to-day by people with disabilities.[1]

Basically, the idea of the ADA was to shore up and protect the civil rights of people with disabilities around employment, education, transportation, telecommunications, and government services.

While noble in nature, the ADA suffered over the years, as the broad definition of the word "disabled" led to protections for people with manageable or invisible symptoms being gradually eroded (for more detail, see "Workplace independence" section in Chapter 7). The law was restored, even improved, when President George W. Bush signed the ADA Amendments Act in 2008. Serving to expand protection to people whose conditions can be mitigated by medications or other means, and refocusing attention on non-discrimination on the basis of even *perceived* disability, the law went into effect on January 1, 2009.

Other federal disability laws that positively changed the lives of many people include: Voting Rights for the Elderly and Handicapped Act (1985), Air Carrier Access Act (1986), and Individuals with Disabilities Education Act (1990), among others.

Gratitude Moment

The next time you take an elevator in a two-story building or park in a designated space on a blazing hot day, think of those who went before us—marching, rolling, limping, shouting, "We *are* important. We *are* part of society. We *are* humans and we have the *right* to be treated with *DIGNITY!*" They are our heroes.

Take a moment. Look at the recent dates on these pieces of legislation. Shake your head in amazement at how things were, and remember that changes such as this don't just happen, but are the result of endless hours of lobbying and activism. Now, send a silent "thank you" to those who opened the doors—and are still holding them open—for us.

Know Your Rights as a Person with Multiple Sclerosis

Until diagnosed with MS, many people may perceive disability rights as those protections offered to people using mobility devices, are blind or hearing-impaired, or coping with other visible "challenges." Once a person feels the impact of MS fatigue, depression, pain, cognitive dysfunction, and other invisible symptoms on their work and daily lives, in most cases he or she probably comes to realize that the disability rights legislation can be leaned on. There are a couple of other documents that are also worth reviewing to remind us of our rights as people with MS in society and our rights as patients in our quest to do the best we can, medically, for ourselves. Although these documents have no binding legal power, they are reminders of how things *should* be in a civilized nation. Referring to the rights enumerated in *The Principles to Promote Quality of Life of People with Multiple Sclerosis* and The Patient's Bill of Rights in your pursuit of dignity and fairness can strengthen your case. These rights should be championed and brought to the forefront of any discussion, whether you are trying to improve the lives of people with MS everywhere by advocating for accessible medications or just trying to get a damn ramp installed at the bathroom of your neighborhood park.

Principles to Promote Quality of Life of People with Multiple Sclerosis

Although the term "human rights" is usually linked with terrible atrocities like genocide happening in far-away places such as East Timor, the whole concept of human rights has a much broader purpose than protecting vulnerable populations from the very worst things that human beings can do to each other. Human rights are about those things that need to happen, or not happen, in order for each person on the planet to live with dignity, simply because they are humans.

As people with multiple sclerosis, we did not become devalued as humans when our immune systems started attacking our myelin and we tired more easily, became less steady on our feet, or slower to find our keys. However, in order for us to live our lives to the fullest and contribute the most we can to society, sometimes we need a little help. We may need special medical care. We may need our workplaces adapted so that we can do our jobs. We may need transportation and public buildings to be made accessible so that we can get where we need to go and function once we get there.

We are not asking for special treatment. We are asking to do the things that humans do. It is in this spirit that the *Principles to Promote Quality of Life of People with Multiple Sclerosis* document was developed by the Multiple Sclerosis International Federation.

The Principles that are specific to people with multiple sclerosis contain many of the rights contained in the United Nations document, *The Declaration on the Rights of Disabled Persons* of December 9, 1975. These "rights," of course, are broad, and there is an explicit acknowledgement that some countries will only be able to "devote limited efforts to this end."

In my opinion, however, it all comes down to this provision in the *Declaration:* "3. Disabled persons have the inherent right to respect for their human dignity. Disabled persons, whatever the origin, nature and seriousness of their handicaps and disabilities, have the same fundamental rights as their fellow-citizens of the same age, which implies first and foremost the right to enjoy a decent life, as normal and full as possible."[2]

The Principles were developed by the authors, then reviewed by a group of experts convened by the MSIF. The authors conducted a series of interviews (with people with MS and doctors) and an extensive literature review, which included journal articles, MS clinical textbooks, and Web-based publications in order to ensure that all relevant points were included.

The introduction to *The Principles* states: "It should always be kept in mind that the ultimate goal is a cure for MS. However, until a cure is found and can be broadly implemented, it is important to work to maintain or improve quality of life for people with MS . . . ."[3] In this context, the term "quality of life" is defined by the World Health Organization as "an individual's perception of their position in life in the context of the culture and value systems in which they live and in relation to their goals, expectations, standards and concerns."

Although they have no legal binding value on their own, *The Principles* were developed so that we, the people living with MS, and those who work to make life better for us (doctors, MS organizations, researchers, governments) have a set of common goals to strive for. This document captures these ideals in one place in the following principles:

1) Independence and empowerment. People with MS are empowered as full participants in their communities and in decision making about the management and treatment of the disease.

2) Medical care. People with MS have access to medical care, treatments, and therapies appropriate to their needs.

3) Continuing (long-term or social) care. People with MS have access to a wide range of age-appropriate care services that enable them to function as independently as possible.

4) Health promotion and disease prevention. People with MS have the information and services they need to maintain positive health practices and a healthy lifestyle.

5) Support for family members. Family members and caregivers receive information and support to mitigate the effects of MS.

6) Transportation. People with MS have access to their communities through accessible public transportation and assistive technology for personal automobiles.

7) Employment and volunteer activities. Support systems and services are available to enable people with MS to continue employment as long as they are productive and desire to work.

8) Disability entitlements and cash assistance. Disability entitlements and services are available to those in need, provide an adequate standard of living, and have flexibility to allow for the disease variability that is characteristic of multiple sclerosis.

9) Education. MS does not inhibit the education of people with MS, their families, or careers.

10) Housing and accessibility of buildings in the community. Accessibility, both of public buildings and in the availability of accessible homes and apartments, is essential to independence for people with MS.

Check Out "The Patient's Bill of Rights"

I guess my favorite document summing up the rights of people entering the medical system is the *Consumer Bill of Rights and Responsibilities* that was adopted by the U.S. Advisory Commission on Consumer Protection and Quality in the Health Care Industry in 1998. It is also known as the "Patient's Bill of Rights." Although these are called "rights," the document itself does not have any legal authority to enforce any of them, but instead states: "The rights enumerated in this report can be achieved in several ways including voluntary actions by health plans, purchasers, facilities, and providers; the effects of market forces; accreditation processes; as well as State or Federal legislation or regulation."[4]

Although not legally binding, "The Patient's Bill of Rights" was created with the right intentions. It was an attempt to give people confidence in the health care system and emphasize the importance of a good relationship between patient and doctor. It also, interestingly enough, laid out the responsibilities of patients to ensure that they were acting as responsible participants in getting the most from their medical care.

The rights contained in the "Patient's Bill of Rights" are summarized as follows:

Information disclosure. You have the right to receive all necessary information about your health plan, doctors and facilities in a format that you can understand so that you can make informed decisions about your health care.

Choice of providers and plans. You have the right to choose the insurance plan and the doctors that are right for your situation.

Access to emergency services. If your health is in immediate danger, you have the right to be stabilized using emergency services without needing to wait for authorization or incurring extra costs.

Participation in treatment decisions. You have the right to know and understand your options for treatment and participate in decisions about your care, as well as be represented by loved ones if you are unable to make these decisions yourself.

Respect and non-discrimination. You have the right to receive respectful, non-discriminatory care from your doctors and insurance representatives.

Confidentiality of health information. You have the right to have your health care information kept protected and confidential. You also have the right to read and copy your own medical record. You have the right to request that incorrect, irrelevant, or incomplete information be changed in your file.

Complaints and appeals. You have the right to a quick and objective review of any complaint you have against your insurance company, doctors and other medical personnel, or facilities. This includes complaints about waiting times and operating hours, how you are treated by medical staff, the adequacy of clinics and hospitals, and other complaints.

Responsibilities as a Person with Multiple Sclerosis

An interesting part of the "Patients' Bill of Rights" is a "Statement of Responsibilities." In a health care system that protects consumers' rights, it is reasonable to expect and encourage consumers to assume reasonable responsibilities. Greater individual involvement by consumers in their care increases the chances that the patients will have a better outcome, that unnecessary costs will be contained, and the system as a whole will function that much better.

Such responsibilities include making an effort to:

- Take responsibility for maximizing healthy habits, such as exercising, not smoking, and eating a healthy diet.

- Become involved in specific health care decisions.

- Work collaboratively with health care providers in developing and carrying out agreed-upon treatment plans.

- Disclose relevant information and clearly communicate wants and needs.

- Use the health plan's internal complaint and appeal processes to address concerns that may arise.

- Recognize the reality of risks and limits of the science of medical care and the human fallibility of the health care professional.

- Be aware of a health care provider's obligation to be reasonably efficient and equitable in providing care to other patients and the community.

- Become knowledgeable about his or her health plan coverage and health plan options (when available) including all covered benefits, limitations, and exclusions, rules regarding use of network providers, coverage and referral rules, appropriate processes to secure additional information, and the process to appeal coverage decisions.

- Show respect for other patients and health workers.

- Make a good-faith effort to meet financial obligations.

- Abide by administrative and operational procedures of health plans, health care providers, and government health benefit programs.

- Report wrongdoing and fraud to appropriate resources or legal authorities.

I find this part of the "Patient's Bill of Rights" interesting—it's almost like a mix between a guide to patient etiquette and a prenuptial agreement between the patient and the health care system. Though I see obvious areas of "CYA" (Cover Your Ass) to provide ethical loopholes for medical professionals and the industry as a whole if abused, many of the points are worth remembering and pursuing in our interactions with the health care system.

Understand the Politics of MS

When considering government politics and policies that impact our lives, and that we might be able to influence in some way, it is important to realize that decisions get made on three levels: federal, state, and city (or local) levels. It is not always immediately clear who is deciding what and what the decision actually means, as states often have loopholes and budgets to allow them to do "their own thing" in many situations. Cities and towns also vary in their implementation of state policy, and even in their adherence to their own regulations, citing budgetary reasons or claiming that an improvement is in the pipeline. Hell, even landlords and owners of individual establishments can avoid complying with code if no one is paying attention. The message here is that you have to dig around to find out what is going on, what the law says, what advocates want to change, who is the target for getting the change made, and how to best reach that person.

Federal Legislation

To find out what is really cooking in terms of active federal legislation around MS, go to GovTrack.us and enter "multiple sclerosis" (in quotation marks) in the Bill Search field. The information there is just as it is described on the Web site:

"GovTrack.us is an independent tool to help the public research and track the activities in the U.S. Congress, promoting government transparency and civic education through novel uses of technology. You'll find here the status of U.S. federal legislation, voting records in the Senate and House of Representatives, and information on Members of Congress, as well as congressional committees and the Congressional Record."

The site also has the full text of all the bills listed. The very best thing about this Web site (at least for me) is that it really explains each step in the process, as well as the terms used. You can truly figure out what is going on and seem really smart after a visit to GovTrack.us. Much of the same information can be found at THOMAS (thomas.loc.gov), a service of the Library of Congress.

Issues on a State or Local Level

Federal policies are important and often determine what happens in our individual lives, but often we are immediately impacted by things regulated on a state level or by our municipal (city or town) governing bodies. Politics surrounding things like affordable housing, accessible transportation, vouchers for respite care, and reducing premiums for state high risk pool insurance may be "hot tickets" at different times in your state or city. You can find out about advocacy specific to people with MS in your area by going to the Web site of your local MS Society chapter. In addition, many issues will be represented by organizations that hold meetings or send out newsletters around the topic and can tell you how you can get involved.

Take Charge

You must understand who has the authority to make a change. Try not to waste your efforts anywhere else.

A Primer of MS Issues

Because we are all individuals with our own unique needs and values, there is no way to provide a comprehensive overview of the issues impacting the lives of everyone with MS. Nevertheless, there are a handful of topics that are pretty specific to MS or could have a considerable impact on the lives of many of us living with the disease. I have pulled together a little primer to help you understand or to remind you of some of the things that MS advocates are calling for at the time of this writing.

Gratitude Moment

An advocate is a person who supports and works toward achieving a specific goal. Lucky for us, there are lots of MS advocates out there. Consider joining them in their fights—they already know the right people and have developed strategies. Add your voice to theirs.

Issue: Lack of National MS Registry

What is the issue and what do advocates want? Estimates of the number of people in the United States living with MS vary widely, from 250,000 to over 500,000. Part of the reason that there is a lack of agreement over the number of cases of MS is that currently, there is not a national coordinated system to collect and analyze data on multiple sclerosis. Not only would such a registry allow for a more accurate estimate of the prevalence and incidence of MS in the United States, it could also provide important epidemiological data about geographic, genetic, and lifestyle factors surrounding MS, as well as give a clearer picture in terms of treatment access and usage. Advocates are calling for support of the National MS and Parkinson's Disease Registries Act (H.R. 1362), a bill that would establish separate Multiple Sclerosis and Parkinson's disease registries at the Agency for Toxic Substances and Disease Registry in the Centers for Disease Control and Prevention (CDC).

How do I find out more or get involved? To find out more, go to the NMSS Web site and type in "MS registry" to see the documents and updates regarding this issue. To read the text of the bill and find out its status, go to GovTrack.us and enter "HR 1362" and "S 1273" in the "Bill Search" field or enter "multiple sclerosis," because the specific bill numbers may change if the bill is amended or during different sessions of Congress.

Issue: Increased Money for MS Research Needed

What is the issue and what do advocates want? The issue is that developing new MS treatments and advancing knowledge around MS requires research, and research requires money. In one "push," the MS Society is requesting that $15 million be allocated to the Congressionally Directed Medical Research Programs (CDMRP) for MS research in 2010, which would mostly go toward investigating a possible link between an increased number of cases of MS and military service. More generally, the MS Society is calling for increased funding to the National Institutes of Health (NIH), namely the National Institute for Neurological Disorders and Stroke. Advocates are also emphasizing the importance of collaboration in research, both among government-funded studies, as well as with the private and non-profit sector, which is an issue close to my heart.

How do I find out more or get involved? Thus far, the MS Society has gotten more than 100,000 people nationwide to sign the petition to increase federal funding for MS research. To find out more, go to the NMSS Web site and click on the menu link to "Government Affairs and Advocacy."

Issue: Representation of People with MS Needed at a Federal Level

What is the issue and what do advocates want? In 2007, the first Congressional Multiple Sclerosis Caucus in the Senate and the House of Representatives was formed. According to the MS Society: "The bi-partisan MS Caucus will serve as a forum for Members of Congress, their staff, related organizations, and individuals to discuss critical health care, disability, research, and other issues affecting people living with MS and other conditions. It will raise awareness and seek creative solutions to help us move closer to a world free of MS."[5]

How do I find out more or get involved? This one is pretty easy. Find out if your legislators have joined and, if not, urge them to join. You can cut to the chase and call your local chapter of the MS Society to find out if your representatives have joined (they will even have the text of a letter for you to sign and send in). Or you can go to Congress.org and find out much more about your individual congressmen and congresswomen and senators, following the links to their individual Web pages and seeing if they are on part of the MS Caucus, among other things. You can also use available forms to write to them electronically.

Make It Better

In some cases, it takes as few as five or ten letters from real people to influence a senator or get his or her attention. Don't underestimate yourself.

Issue: Restricted Access to Private Insurance and Other Issues Around Affordable Health Care

What is the issue and what do advocates want? Currently, those of us with MS can be denied health coverage by insurance carriers, which use "pre-existing conditions" as a way of turning people down who apply for policies. This has several ramifications. Some of us stay in jobs that we dislike or that are too physically demanding for fear that we will be unable to get or afford health insurance coverage if we leave our current employer. Those of us who have to leave jobs, are self-employed, or were never covered, end up in the position of not having health insurance at all or paying far higher premiums to our state's "high-risk pool" insurance, which carries high deductibles (my deductible is $5,000) and premiums costing double the regular private insurance. Needless to say, there are many implications for this, as people end up unable to afford health care or limit utilization to save money. Advocates want guaranteed eligibility, whereby health insurance companies would have to approve anyone, regardless of health condition. Small business owners and the self-employed would also be protected. Opponents of this idea say that there is no way that private insurance companies can afford to take care of the "traditionally uninsurable," and that this will cause a collapse of the current system.

Besides guaranteed eligibility for private health insurance, there are many ways to get to the idea of health coverage for everyone. Each strategy has pros and cons, as well as people who say their idea is the *only* solution, whereas others say it would *never* work. There are groups calling for limiting payment to cover only things recommended by a committee who would evaluate current practices and put out standards for evidence-based medicine. There are groups saying that Medicaid should increase the cutoff for income eligibility to several times the FLP (federal poverty level). Others advocate lower premiums for the state high-risk pools. Others call for a single-payer system of universal health care.

How do I find out more or get involved? These are just a few of the proposed ideas to work toward accessible health care—each of the ideas has its own advocacy groups and supporters. A good place to start learning about these issues is Families USA (www.familiesusa .org), an organization that touts itself as "The Voice for Health Care Consumers." The Web site contains tons of information about the different issues and approaches to reaching "health equity," as well as links to individual state pages listing advocacy organizations in each state and news about the various health coverage issues in each state.

Issue: Need for Affordable Access to Specialty Drugs and Examination of "Tier" Classification System

What is the issue and what do advocates want? In insurance formularies, drugs are classified into four tiers, with most drugs in the following three tiers: $5 generic, $10 or more for preferred-brand, and $25 or more for non-preferred brands. Specialty drugs, such as disease-modifying therapies for MS, reside at the far end of the spectrum in Tier 4. A couple things are happening here. Insurance companies are starting to charge a percentage (20% to 33%) of drug costs for Tier 4 drugs, rather than the usual fixed-amount co-pay. As MS disease-modifying drugs can cost upwards of $2,500 per month, this arrangement puts these medications out of financial reach for many people. Financial burden is also increased as insurers reclassify certain drugs (especially ones being used off-label) to higher tiers, which allows them to increase the co-pay. Some journalists and advocates are claiming that the Tier 4 classification is saved for drugs for rare diseases because the number of people affected by this system is too small for them to organize and demand change. At this point, advocates want legislation to make the process around drug pricing and tier classification more transparent. In some states, senators are moving to banish the Tier 4 classification altogether.

How do I find out more or get involved? One way to find out more is to enter "tier 4 drugs multiple sclerosis" in your search engine to see all the most recent news articles. To find out what is happening in your area, go to the Web site of your chapter of the NMSS and enter "tier 4 drugs" in the search box or call the chapter to find out what is happening with this issue.

Issue: 24-Month Medicare Waiting Period

What is the issue and what do advocates want? Under the current system, there is a two-year waiting period before people can receive any healthcare coverage through Medicare. It is estimated that 1.5 million people are living with disabilities that prevent them from working, and qualify for Social Security disability benefits. An estimated 39% of these people are left without health insurance at some point during this two-year waiting period, because they cannot afford COBRA or don't qualify for private health insurance. This leads to either extreme financial hardships as people try to pay out-of-pocket, or forgo medical care altogether. What advocates want is pretty simple: the elimination of any waiting period and for Medicare to be available at the same time disability benefits are awarded.

How do I find out more or get involved? For more information, go to the MS Society Web site and click the "Advocacy" link. You can also go to GovTrack.us and search for "S 700" or "HR 1708," or Google "Ending the Medicare Disability Waiting Period Act of 2009.

More Controversial Topics

Issue: Restrictions on Embryonic Stem-Cell Research

What is the issue and what do advocates want? The stem cell controversy is the ethical debate about doing research on (thus destroying) human embryos to create embryonic stem cell lines. The main opposition to this type of research has its root in the idea that human life begins at conception; thus, to the opponents of stem cell research, destroying these embryos is tantamount to murder. Opponents also point out that there are already several medical advances and treatments using adult stem cells, whereas embryonic stem cells have yet to yield anything currently in use. Advocates of embryonic stem cell research claim that there are hundreds of thousands of embryos left over from in vitro fertilization procedures; therefore new embryos would not have to be "created," but scientists could use embryos that were eventually going to be destroyed anyway. Stem cell therapy has already shown great potential to treat multiple sclerosis and advocates claim that limitations on embryonic stem cell research is slowing down access to potentially life-changing treatments.

This issue is slightly outdated, because on March 9, 2009, President Barack Obama removed certain restrictions on federal funding for research involving new lines of human embryonic stem cells. Prior to this order being signed, federal funding was limited to non-embryonic stem cell research and embryonic stem cell research based upon embryonic stem cell lines already in existence, although private funding has never been prohibited.

How do I find out more or get involved? There is a ton of information about stem cell research on the Internet. Since the lifting of the biggest legislative barrier to embryonic stem cell research, advocates have turned their attention to wondering "Why isn't it going faster?" and "Why don't I have access to stem cell treatment that is showing promise in other countries?"

> ### Know Your Stuff
>
> To be an effective advocate, you need to learn about both sides of an issue. Be able to debate both sides. This will enable you to explain your views much better and will make your arguments much more convincing.

Issue: Medical Marijuana Remains Illegal in Most States

What is the issue and what do advocates want? In most states of the United States, the possession and growing of marijuana is illegal. Although a number of states have recognized medical marijuana as a viable treatment (14 at the time of this writing), only California, New Mexico and Rhode Island have "operationalized" the idea by having dispensaries that sell it. (Several countries allow for medical use of marijuana, including Canada, Austria, the Netherlands, Spain, Israel, Finland, and Portugal.) However, marijuana is touted by many people with MS (and other health issues) as the only thing that helps many of their symptoms. It is also inexpensive and it has few side effects. Research into medical marijuana is generally positive, although some data shows that it is detrimental to cognitive function and coordination issues in people with MS. Its usefulness is acknowledged by several professional associations, including the American Medical Association, the Institute of Medicine, and the National Academy of Science. The bottom line is that people want medical marijuana to be legal. Ideally, it would also be made easily available with a prescription, but many advocates would be happy if they were just given permission to grow it themselves.

How do I find out more or get involved? There are several organizations that have taken on the fight for the legalization of medical marijuana. Americans for Safe Access (www.safeaccessnow.org) is "the nation's largest organization of patients, medical professionals, scientists, and concerned citizens promoting safe and legal access to cannabis for therapeutic use and research." The Web site contains both medical and legal information, as well as forums. There are a number of opportunities to get involved as an activist on different levels, including organizing your own group, sending online letters and petitions, interacting with the media, and communicating with government representatives.

Other organizations advocating for the legalization of medical marijuana include: Marijuana Policy Project (www.mpp.org), The National Organization for the Reform of Marijuana Laws/NORML (www .norml.org), and The Drug Policy Alliance (www.drugpolicy.org).

Issue: Assisted Suicide Remains Illegal

What is the issue and what do advocates want? Otherwise known as "euthanasia," this practice involves physicians administering a lethal combination of drugs to a person who wishes to die because they feel that they no longer have a good quality of life and are suffering. In most countries of the world, including 44 states of the United States, assisted suicide is illegal. Opponents claim that it goes against the Hippocratic Oath that doctors take to "do no harm." Many people also maintain that the application of assisted suicide is too difficult to control and could easily be used to "kill" people that have become burdens to their loved ones or by people who are mentally unstable and may not be fully aware of the implications or who have the chance to recover. It also goes against the teachings of many major religions.

Advocates claim that assisted suicide is a matter of freedom of choice. They claim that the option to "die with dignity" is a human right. Advocates with MS want this option available to them in case their disability progresses to the point that they feel that they no longer wish to live in a state of total dependence on others.

How do I find out more or get involved? It is a little difficult to recommend sites with unbiased information about assisted suicide, as the majority are either very supportive of the idea or morally opposed to it. For this reason, I recommend starting with the "Euthanasia" page of ProCon.org (www.procon.org), a non-profit organization that claims: "We promote critical thinking, education, and informed citizenship. Our sites present controversial issues in a straightforward, nonpartisan, primarily pro-con format." The site nicely lays out the debate on both sides, including the positions of the various world religions, individual state laws, and international perspectives.

Be an Activist

For all of the unpredictability and heartbreak that is part of the multiple sclerosis package, we are truly fortunate to have strong organizations behind us. My friend with lupus complains that there is not a cohesive "lupus community" like we have, she feels that no one is advocating for people with lupus and that it is one of those diseases that people rarely hear about. Indeed, it is pretty cool that we can just decide one day to get involved as an activist for our cause and a whole catalogue of opportunities opens up to us via these organizations.

The National Multiple Sclerosis Society (NMSS) is the giant who "has our back" as people with MS. The NMSS has formal activist and volunteer programs set up across the country, giving us the opportunity to either jump right in to full-fledged lobbying or get our feet wet by assisting with education campaigns or fundraising events. There are other organizations, MS-specific and focused on other issues, that would also welcome our voices and participation with open arms.

Take Charge

Be an activist. Direct your frustration into effectively making things better.

MS Activist Network

Not only is the National Multiple Sclerosis Society raising money for research and client programs, a large component of their activities is activism. They have done a great job of organizing the logistics and creating an infrastructure to allow anyone to take on advocacy at the level that they are comfortable with through the MS Activist Network. When you join the MS Activist Network, you will be given information and tools to allow you to confidently address the issues important to people with MS, and alerted via "MS Action Alerts" and monthly e-newsletters about critical moments needing your participation, as well as successes and future campaigns.

Make It Better

Although many people think of activists as those people who are screaming, protesting, and resisting arrest to get a point across, I have a broader definition. I think an activist is anyone who puts effort toward making things better in the world. Activists are people who lick envelopes, who hold strangers' hands, who deliver meals.

Whether you are more of a "screamer" or an "envelope licker," get involved. We need all the help we can get.

Some of the ways that the MS Activist Network encourages people to get involved include:

Meet with public officials, such as members of Congress. You can make an appointment or just stop in to discuss an issue important to you with members of Congress in your local district. To find out who these people are, you can go to Congress.org and enter your zip code. You can find their contact information this way and call their office to find out when they might be in town. You can also find out when your legislator will hold town hall meetings.

Write a letter to the editor. This is a good way to get people interested in an issue, especially if you have a personal story to support your point. This is a good forum to call people to perform a specific action. Pointers from the MS Society include: "Write a persuasive letter, be thoughtful and polite. Be sure to ask for the action you want. And be brief. Editors are most likely to publish a letter no longer than 150–250 words. Remember to include your full name and address."

Call into a radio talk show. The MS Society suggests the following: "Write out what you want to say beforehand. Then keep dialing until you get through. When you do, share your story and be positive. Be clear and concise about the point you want to make. Don't engage in argument. Say what you want to say, then hang up."

Other Opportunities to Take Action

Maybe you want to do something, but aren't sure that hanging out with politicians or lobbying on "the Hill" is for you. You can check out some additional opportunities to help by starting with a search on VolunteerMatch.com. They cooperate with many non-profit organizations to help you find opportunities in your geographic area. They also list volunteer opportunities that are "virtual," meaning that you could do them from home.

Some of the opportunities that came up when I did a search are less about lobbying and more about helping people in a more direct way. They included:

MS Ambassadors and Speakers Bureau. A program of the NMSS, the MS Ambassador program is described as follows: "The National MS

Society is looking for people who are passionate about spreading awareness of Multiple Sclerosis and the different programs and services the Society has to offer. MS Ambassadors will serve as the "face" of the Society and will spread awareness within their community by attending college fairs, speaking at schools, various clubs; basically anywhere more information about MS is desired." You can also sign up to be a part of the local Speaker's Bureau to speak to healthcare providers and other interested community groups about MS.

Consider some of these other volunteer opportunities:

Peer counselors and mentors. Peer counselors are trained volunteers who provide phone counseling to people with MS from their own homes. There are also "newly diagnosed mentors" to help people who have just received a diagnosis of MS. MS Angel Visitors are people who visit people with MS in their homes or in care facilities. These are programs of NMSS, which can vary by chapter.

MSFriends is an organization that runs a 24-hour-a-day helpline, which is staffed with trained volunteers with MS who operated under the guiding motto of "friends helping friends." They are looking for peer support volunteers with MS who have at least two years of experience working with people with MS as a support volunteer or in a medical capacity, have a basic knowledge of MS, and are able to volunteer five hours per week. To find out more, visit www.msfriends.org or call 1-866-msfriends (1-866-673-7436).

Information and referral specialists. These are trained volunteers at individual NMSS chapters who answer calls from clients and their family members or caretakers to answer questions about MS, as well as provide information about services and insurance.

LINCS (Linking Individuals in Need with Care and Services) volunteer counselors. This is a program of the Medicare Rights Center that trains volunteers to help people navigate the Medicare system, including determining eligibility and filling out forms and applications. Volunteers provide this help by phone from their own homes. To find out more about this program, contact the LINCS Program Coordinators at 212-204-6273 or e-mail LINCS@medicarerights.org.

In Your Own Backyard

Changing the world for the better does not require millions of dollars or a big infrastructure. As we go through life, opportunities to help someone or improve things will present themselves—especially if we keep our eyes open.

For instance, do you have a hard time getting your wheelchair into the local movie theater? Sure, it is easy to find another activity or stay home and rent another DVD of the movie you want to see. But our lives get limited enough when we are beset by physical symptoms beyond our control—any accessibility problem that further "clips our wings" is unacceptable, not only for our full enjoyment of what life has to offer, but also for other people in similar situations. Write a letter to the theater owners and see what happens. If the response is not to your satisfaction, call up your local newspaper or write a letter to the editor. Keep in mind that most cities have a dedicated person, called an ADA Coordinator, to ensure that establishments are compliant with the Americans with Disabilities Act (ADA). Call "311" to get the information about who this person is in your city and how to contact her or him. Open up the door for yourself and others.

Fundraising Opportunities

One easy way to get "your feet wet" in getting involved with organizations helping people is to help raise money for these organizations so they can continue their work. It is a good way to meet people and make friends with an interest in MS, or another issue close to your heart, as well as to scope out the organization and get a feel for it before getting more involved. Here are a couple of ways that you can offer support:

Participate in an event or support an event. These days it seems like people don't really *just* write checks. Instead, they ride their bicycles 150 miles, walk or run various distances, golf, dance, or do all sorts of other things to raise money. If you are physically up to the challenge, participating in one of these events can be really fun and a great way to remind yourself of the effort that people are putting in to support MS research and programs (although many people participate for the sheer physical challenge and have little interest in the benefitting organization). Especially when it comes to MS fundraising events, there are usually provisions to ensure that people in wheelchairs and using mobility devices can participate. If you are not overly excited about the idea of riding a bicycle for two days uphill, there are usually plenty of opportunities to volunteer to support the event participants or assist with logistics, both leading up to and on event day. Your help will be hugely appreciated if you are willing to do "boring" tasks, such as stuff envelopes or compile packets of information for participants.

Do Your Best

You can always adapt a sporting event. For instance, some MSers ride in the MS bike tours with a group on stationary bikes so they don't overheat. Find a substitute (but equivalent) activity for fundraising that you can do, and go out and tell people about it.

Volunteer to help with fundraising. Some organizations and chapters have well-run volunteer programs and will be thrilled to let you do something to raise money or raise awareness, such as send out preprinted letters requesting donations or staff a booth at a big gathering.

Hold your own event to raise money for your favorite organization. This can be a really fun thing to do to help fundraise for an organization. Pretty much the "sky's the limit" in terms of thinking about what kind of event to hold. You can have a simple cocktail party for a small number of people, during which you speak about your own experience with MS and ask for a donation. Or you can put together a large picnic and invite people from your church to bring food. You can get together with your friends and hold a bake sale, a bowling tournament, or a garage sale, with the proceeds going to your favorite organization. It is very important to let people who you invite to participate, especially in the social events, know that this is a fundraiser and they will be asked for money—this can help avoid any awkwardness around "making the ask."

For young people. There are a couple of opportunities specifically for young people interested in getting involved with MS advocacy and fundraising. One is YAMS, which stands for Youth Against Multiple Sclerosis (youthagainstms.org). It was founded by two 13-year-olds in 2000, one of whom had just been diagnosed with MS. The organization primarily coordinates teams for MS walks, as well as holds educational workshops in schools to teach young people about MS. YAMS also maintains a Web site and sends out a newsletter three times per year.

Another opportunity for young people to get involved is to participate in the MS Leadership Development Program, a paid internship program for college students at Bayer HealthCare's U.S. Headquarters in Wayne, New Jersey. Interns are exposed to different aspects of public policy and advocacy, as well as the marketing and patient relations side of the business. To learn more, go to www.multiplesclerosis.com/internships.

The Bottom Line

When many people hear the words "advocacy" or "activism," they picture people screaming and holding placards, fighting for the right to life, the right to choose, the rights of prisoners not to die, the rights of the terminally ill to assisted suicide, or some other life-or-death cause.

Activism around health issues exploded into the public eye in the United States at the beginning of the AIDS crisis in this country. Everyone was very frightened of this new disease, blame was everywhere, and people simply did not know what to do. People were divided in their views, and in many cases, discrimination deepened. In the 20-plus years since the virus first made an appearance in the United States, think how far we have come.

To remind you of the desperation of a nation and marginalization and fear of some of the people in it, take a journey back in time and read what Vito Russo had to say over two decades ago in a speech in front of the Department of Health and Human Services during a demonstration on Monday, October 10, 1988, called "Why We Fight":

> " . . . I wanted to speak out today as a person with AIDS who is not dying. You know, for the last three years, since I was diagnosed, my family thinks two things about my situation. One, they think I'm going to die, and two, they think that my government is doing absolutely everything in their power to stop that. And they're wrong, on both counts . . . .

> And it's worse than a war, because during a war people are united in a shared experience. This war has not united us, it's divided us. It's separated those of us with AIDS and those of us who fight for people with AIDS from the rest of the population

. . . they don't spend their waking hours going from hospital room to hospital room, and watching the people that they love die slowly—of neglect and bigotry, because it isn't happening to them and they don't have to give a shit. They haven't been to two funerals a week for the last three or four or five years—so they don't give a shit, because it's not happening to them . . . .

Someday, the AIDS crisis will be over. Remember that. And when that day comes—when that day has come and gone, there'll be people alive on this earth—gay people and straight people, men and women, black and white, who will hear the story that once there was a terrible disease in this country and all over the world, and that a brave group of people stood up and fought and, in some cases, gave their lives, so that other people might live and be free . . . ."[6]

Vito Russo died two years later, on November 7, 1990, from AIDS-related complications. Having lived in Greenwich Village during this era, I still cannot read that speech and not get tears in my eyes. It really was like this.

Two decades later, things are different for all of us with health problems, including those of us living with multiple sclerosis. Besides people with MS, many other individuals who may have once kept information and fears about their illness to themselves out of embarrassment or fear of being misunderstood have found their voices and come together to speak up and speak out. These include, among others, cancer survivors, people with mental illness, and parents of children with disabilities. They demand equality, inclusion in society, that resources be directed toward research, that the flaws in the health care system be remedied, and that they be allowed to live with dignity.

In his book that profiles five people living with different chronic illnesses, *Strong at the Broken Places*, Richard Cohen says calmly, but firmly, "These are the faces of illness in America. Do not look away. The characters may surprise you, even shatter a stereotype or two. They are people, not cases, survivors, not victims."[7]

As people, as survivors, we *can* make a big difference, especially if we work together. We can make a difference for ourselves and for those who cannot speak for themselves. We can be strengthened in our shared experience and make this experience the very best it can be.

Conclusion: The *Bottom* Bottom Line

As I sit here typing these final words, it is currently 103 degrees where I live. I wanted to complete writing this book before it got hot and my brain shut down. I *almost* made it.

I have come a long way since first receiving my diagnosis and suffering through my first anxiety-filled Solu-Medrol "trip." I am an old pro at giving myself daily injections of Copaxone, and I am becoming increasingly convinced that my personal experiment with low-dose naltrexone is making a difference in my quality of life. I still cry and rage about the injustice of MS, for myself and for others living with this disease—however, my sadness has taken on a more mature quality than the original "Why me?" sniffling I used to indulge in. I no longer feel the need to talk about every symptom I am experiencing to everyone I meet in minute detail; I have learned that the subject quickly becomes tiresome—especially to me. Oh, I still bitch about my MS to whomever will listen, but I have found that laughing about it at times can also be a salve on the wounds.

I am squinting out my window at the shimmers of the heat outside and hoping that I have done justice to my mission of holding out a hand to pull readers out of MS quicksand, letting you know there are shoulders to cry on and friends to be made. I am sure that in several years I will read parts of this book and think to myself, "Wow. What was I thinking when I wrote *that?*" However, I shared from the heart. My wish is that your truth maps on to mine in places and that I cleared a couple of rocks out of your path. Thank you for giving me this opportunity.

Take care of yourselves, my friends.

Appendix
National Multiple Sclerosis Society Resources

My Life, My MS, My Decisions

http://www.nationalMSsociety.org/mylifemymsmydecisions

Online classes to help people boost their decision-making power.

- Teaming Up with Your Healthcare Providers
- Navigating the Medication Maze
- Considering Clinical Trials
- Achieving Optimal Wellness

Self-Advocacy materials

http://www.nationalMSsociety.org/selfadvocacy

These materials describe effective practices and communication styles people can use to represent themselves and their interests in important areas of everyday life. They also provide resources, tools and templates for becoming a more effective self-advocate.

- Self-advocacy for health insurance, appeals and Medicare issues
  http://www.nationalMSsociety.org/selfadvocacyinsurance
- Self-advocacy and employment
  http://www.nationalMSsociety.org/selfadvocacyemployment
- Self-advocacy for medical care and long-term care
  http://www.nationalMSsociety.org/selfadvocacymedical

- Self-advocacy and Social Security Disability Insurance
  http://www.nationalMSsociety.org/selfadvocacySSDI

- Self-advocacy in the family environment
  http://www.nationalMSsociety.org/selfadvocacyfamily

- Self-advocacy in the community
  http://www.nationalMSsociety.org/selfadvocacycommunity

Workplace Disclosure Tool

http://www.nationalMSsociety.org/disclosuretool

The decision to disclose personal medical information in the workplace is a complex one, requiring careful thought and planning. So it's important for people to weigh their options carefully before making a decision to disclose—keeping in mind that once information is given, it can never be taken back.

Multimedia Library

http://www.nationalMSsociety.org/multimedialibrary

Brochures, online videos, DVDs, Webcasts, podcasts related to the diagnosis, management, and lifestyle challenges of MS.

MyMSMyWay.com

www.MyMSMyWay.com

MyMSMyWay is a free resource dedicated to connecting those living with MS to accessible technologies that can help them live their lives better. The site was developed by the MS Technology Collaborative, a landmark alliance of organizations passionate about helping people with multiple sclerosis (MS) maximize their abilities.

Relationship Matters: A Program for Couples Living with MS

http://www.nationalMSsociety.org/relationshipmatters

This program, funded by a grant from the United States Department of Health and Human Services, Administration for Children and Families, can help couples strengthen their partnership and minimize the impact of MS on their lives. Through a series of in-person, teleconference and online options, couples learn techniques and information to keep their most important relationships moving forward.

Financial Planning Resources

http://www.nationalMSsociety.org/financialplanning

Resources to begin planning financially for the future, including evaluating your income, assets, debts, benefits, and other resources is essential to being well-prepared for a future with MS:

- *Adapting: Financial Planning for a Life with Multiple Sclerosis*—A free 72-page book that addresses financial organization, planning, insurance options, employment concerns, and benefit issues important to people with MS and their families.
- Through the Financial Education Partners (FEP) program, people with MS and their families can access free financial counseling and education from members of the Society of Financial Service Professionals by calling 1-800-344-4867, option 1.

National MS Society Financial Assistance Program

http://www.nationalMSsociety.org/financialassistance

The Society's Financial Assistance program offers guidance, support and resources to help contain the financial impact of MS.

Social Security Disability

http://www.nationalMSsociety.org/socialsecuritydisability

Information and materials designed to guide people through the application process for Social Security Disability benefits, including a set of guidebooks for people with MS and their physicians.

Keep S'myelin

http://www.nationalMSsociety.org/ks

A colorful, engaging, informative, and reassuring newsletter to help children 6-12 and their parents talk and learn about MS together. Available online in an interactive version or a print version, or by mail by calling 1-800-344-4867, option 1.

References

Chapter 1

1. Prince SD. (ed.) 1001 Smartest Things Ever Said. Guilford: Lyons Press, 2004: 14.

2. Bandura A. Self-efficacy. In: Ramachaudran VS, ed. Encyclopedia of human behavior. New York: Academic Press, 1994: vol. 4, 71–81.

Chapter 2

1. Healthy People 2010. Home Page. Retrieved from: http: //www.healthy people.gov.

2. Atlas of MS Database. Retrieved from: http: //www.atlasofms.org.

3. McDonald WI, Compston A, Edan G, et al.. Recommended diagnostic criteria for multiple sclerosis: Guidelines from the International Panel on the diagnosis of multiple sclerosis. *Annals of Neurology.* 2001; 50(1), 121–7.

4. Polman CH, Reingold SC, Edan G, et al. Diagnostic criteria for multiple sclerosis: 2005 revisions to the "McDonald Criteria." *Annals of Neurology,* 2005; 58(6): 840–6.

5. Stachowiak J. Multiple Sclerosis Relapses. Retrieved from http:// ms.about.com.

6. Poser CM, Paty DW, Scheinber L, et al. New Diagnostic Criteria for Multiple Sclerosis; Guidelines for Research Protocols. *Annals of Neurology,* 1983; 13(3); 227–231.

Chapter 3

1. American Psychiatric Association 2000. (DSM-IV-TR) Diagnostic and statistical manual of mental disorders, 4th edition, text revision. Washington, DC: American Psychiatric Press, Inc., 2000.

2. Gingold JN. Facing the Cognitive Challenges of Multiple Sclerosis. New York: Demos Medical Publishing, 2006.

Chapter 4

1. Minden SL, Hoaglin DC, Hadden L, et al. Access to and utilization of neurologists by people with multiple sclerosis. *Neurology*, 2008; 70, (13), 1141–1149.

2. Groopman, J. How Doctors Think. New York: Mariner Books, 2007.

Chapter 5

1. Birnbaum G, Cree B, Altafullah I, et al. Combining beta interferon and atorvastatin may increase disease activity in multiple sclerosis. *Neurology*, 2008; 71(18), 1390–5.

2. Costello K, Kennedy P, Scanzillo J. Recognizing nonadherence in patients with multiple sclerosis and maintaining treatment adherence in the long term. The *Medscape Journal of Medicine*, 2008; 10(9). 225.

Chapter 6

1. Olsen, SA. A review of complementary and alternative medicine (CAM) by people with multiple sclerosis. *Occupational Therapy International*, 2009; 16(1), 57–70.

2. Loren MF, Phil B, and Small E. Yoga and Multiple Sclerosis: A Journey to Health and Healing. New York: Demos Health, 2007.

3. Bowling, AC. Complementary and Alternative Medicine and Multiple Sclerosis. 2nd ed. New York: Demos Health, 2007.

Chapter 7

1. Rumrill, PD. Employment Issues and Multiple Sclerosis. 2nd ed. New York: Demos Medical Publishing, 2008.

2. Joffe R, Friedlander J. Women, Work, and Autoimmune Disease: Keep Working, Girlfriend! New York: Demos Health, 2008.

3. Karp, G. Life on Wheels: The A to Z Guide to Living Fully with Mobility Issues. New York: Demos Health, 2008.

Chapter 8

1. Preamble to the Constitution of the World Health Organization as adopted by the International Health Conference, New York, 19–22 June, 1946.

2. Russell, RD. Social Health: An Attempt to Clarify This Dimension of Well-Being. *International Journal of Health Education*, 1973; 16, 74–82.

3. Pollan, M. In Defense of Food: An Eater's Manifesto. New York: The Penguin Group, 2008.

4. Zhang L, Samet J, Caffo B, et al. Cigarette Smoking and Nocturnal Sleep Architecture. *American Journal of Epidemiology*, 2006; 164(6), 529–537.

Chapter 10

1. Gladwell, M. Blink: The Power of Thinking Without Thinking. New York: Little, Brown and Company, 2005.

2. Edwards, L. Life Disrupted: Getting Real About Chronic Illness in Your Twenties and Thirties. New York: Walker and Company, 2008.

3. Isaksson AK, Gunnarsson LG and Ahlström G. The presence and meaning of chronic sorrow in patients with multiple sclerosis. *Journal of Clinical Nursing*, 2007; 16(11C), 315–324.

4. Gleason, T. MS emotions: Anger. Multiple Sclerosis Blog of September 8, 2006. Retrieved from: www.everydayhealth.com/blog/trevis-life-with-multiple-sclerosis-ms.

5. Mohr DC, Dick LP, Russo D, et al. The psychosocial impact of multiple sclerosis: exploring the patient's perspective. *Health Psychology*; 1999; 18(4), 376–382.

Chapter 11

1. Salon (gathering) Wikipedia entry. Retrieved from: http://en.wikipedia.org/wiki/Literary_salon.

Chapter 12

1. Americans with Disabilities Act of 1990, Pub. L. No. 101–336, §2, 104 Stat. 328; 1991.

2. United Nations General Assembly. Declaration on the Rights of Disabled Persons, G.A. res. 3447 (XXX), 30 U.N. GAOR Supp. (No. 34) at 88, U.N. Doc. A/10034; 1975.

3. Multiple Sclerosis International Foundation. Principles to Promote the Quality of Life of People with MS, 2005. Retrieved from: http://www .msif.org/en/resources/msif_resources/msif_publications/quality_of_life _principles/index.html.

4. President's Advisory Committee on Consumer Protection and Quality in the Health Care Industry. Consumer Bill of Rights and Responsibilities, 1997. Retrieved from: http://www.hcqualitycommission.gov/cborr.

5. Announcing New Congressional MS Caucus. I'm an MS Activist blog. Monday, July 23, 2007. Retrieved from: http://msactivist.blogspot.com/ 2007_07_01_archive.html.

6. Russo V. Transcript of speech "Why We Fight." ACT UP Demonstration at the Department of Health and Human Services, Washington D.C. October 10, 1988.

7. Cohen, RM. Strong at the Broken Places: Voices of Illness, a Chorus of Hope. New York: Harper Collins Publisher, 2008.

Index

Note: Throughout this index, the abbreviation MS is used for multiple sclerosis.